TRAPPED: THE WAY OU...

A YOGIC GUIDE TOWARDS HEALING

THE BEGINNERS GUIDE TO SELF DISCOVERY

BY JAMEL RANDALL

Trapped: The Way Out Is Within:
A Yogic Guide Toward Healing
Copyright © 2022 Jamel Randall. All Rights Reserved.

For more information about this title or to order other books
and/or electronic media, contact the publisher:

ISBN
979-8-9872955-0-2 (Paperback)
979-8-9872955-2-6 (eBook)

Printed in the United States of America

Cover and Interior design: Van-garde Imagery

Contents

Preface

YEARS AGO, I found myself in the center of a yoga studio surrounded by about 30-40 people, mostly white and definitely only women. *Downward Dog,* is the pose the class patiently waited for me to get into, but I had no clue what a Down Dog was. My cover was blown. I confessed.

"Hey, I'm gonna be honest with y'all. I lied about being experienced in yoga. I just wanted to get accepted into the training."

My teacher smiled at me.

"Jamel, we smelled your bullshit weeks ago. I'm glad you finally came out of your shell and told us the truth. The practice is much greater than the physical postures. So the only thing you need to be accepted in the training is who you are today. Remember, no level of improvement can outweigh self-acceptance."

Those words would churn me down the road of self-discovery. A journey of freeing myself through self acceptance.

One of the most polarizing reference points throughout my training was the yoga sutras written by the sage Patanjali Jois. Living in the inner city of Detroit, my story sounds different, but the perspective still had great relevance. The scripture contains the famous eight limbs of yoga. These limbs reflect the natural capabilities within us, and the means toward unfolding these limbs lead to overall enlightenment.

Enlightenment that can lead to remarkable personal growth, regardless of culture or religious background. This book is an endeavor intended to present an effective and relatable perspective on yoga philosophy and mindset in an easy-to-read book anyone can use along their journey towards self-enlightenment.

The center of all progress lies within the core of each human's personal desires. When time-tested methods for stimulating the process of transformation are applied intentionally, remarkable progress can occur within any cultural or religious setting. Anyone who has the desire can build a daily practice routine for the long term, leading to the steady cultivation of enlightenment in everyday life.

In this book, we go from a centuries-old philosophy and translate it into a modern city perspective. It's amazing how far apart culture, age, race, and other circumstances can be while still having a denominator of commonality.

The stories I tell throughout this book are my humble attempt to shine a light on how the lessons and practice of yoga helped me find liberation when I was at my darkest.

Yoga guided me through an extremely rough patch of life, and I've found a purpose in sharing this light. I've shared my story with thousands, and I've listened to the stories of many. There's power within opening yourself up to experience life in its totality, not just the comfortable parts.

In fact, a major part of my healing journey is being vulnerable enough to write this book. There is an extreme discomfort in placing words to pages and leaving it for others to process. My comfort zone is being able to convince you to see what I am saying from my point of view. Yet I understand that the joy of books is the many perspectives that come from reading.

The stories that I share within these pages unveil the steps toward living a life free from hesitation and doubt. So many allow their fears and doubts to prevent them from even attempting to live out their greatest dreams. This method is a clear and direct guide to just begin. I call it the TRAP method:

Trusting in your today. Trusting that life happens for you, instead of against you.

Revealing your story to relinquish your attachment to the past. This not only frees you, but it also inspires others. Think of the generations of secrets kept by our ancestors who were looking to protect us by withholding the truth. The embarrassment of exposing weak abusers leaves a generation feeling they are all alone. The fact is, none of us are alone. Yes, abuse is a gruesome level of withholding the truth, but as you read along, you discover that this relates to all levels of life. I can't keep count of the many students who come into my yoga studio who fear being seen as inflexible or unstable. Essentially afraid to expose their truth. We will discover how being vulnerable on your yoga mat will open you up to being vulnerable and standing powerfully in your truth off the mat.

Acceptance in who you are now because no level of improvement can ever outweigh self-acceptance. Still, setting your **A**im as growth is the key toward continued happiness. We must set an aim within everything we do in life, or else we will go through the motions, unaware of where we have come and where we are going.

Practice over **P**erfection. The motto that was cemented into my brain as a child was "practice makes perfect." Well, after years of trying this out, I've witnessed that perfection is not attainable—and even if it were, the pressure and sacrifices of precious moments in life make it not worth it. I want to encourage you to take the mindset of practice over perfection. The yoga lessons that you will learn in this book will tie into the way you approach everything in life.

People have widely seen yoga as a practice of stretching and breathing. Some may naturally tie deeper meaning to it, such as it is a way to find peace and clarity. These are both accurate statements; however, the more transformative perspective of yoga is this: *Yoga provides a lens to see within. Through the postures and breath, you can observe everything that defines who you are currently.*

The way you respond to what you see determines your peace. The aim is for you to develop the mindset of acceptance and detachment from both the good and bad things that come up in life.

I would be remiss if I hadn't cut a space to acknowledge the contributors to my life's perspective, beginning with my football coaches. Although they coached me as a child, it wasn't until I came back out to coach the Detroit Broncos as a 19-year-old adult that I appreciated and understood the gems they've always implanted into not just me but the entire community.

Next would be my yoga teacher, Jonny Kest. Never did I expect a white guy from Birmingham, Michigan to be one of the greatest influences in my life, but boy, you are that. Your light and perspective on life is a gift to the world, and I am forever grateful that you viewed me as a vessel to continue to spread the practice of yoga to my community. Last but not least, my parents. The silent lessons you taught me continue to expose themselves with each passing year since your death. It was a traumatic time in my life to have both parents pass in consecutive years, but as life continues to unfold, I realize the resilience that I have gained by being a witness to the unavoidable cycle of life.

This book is merely a hello for the readers. This series of books, titled "Trapped," should make life more digestible. The mindful practices that have allowed me to find liberation and peace within gloomy times of life. A voice to a community that isn't always reached. A perspective on life that isn't told in this light.

We all have a story. It's our perspective that will determine how we tell it. Make sure when it's your time to share, it is a true, raw and unafraid authentic truth. I'm looking forward to being your tour guide along the way.

Part 1: Mindful Visions Framework

As YOU WILL learn in this book, the aim in a yoga practice is to use the postures to see within. The way you respond to discomfort in a posture. How do you sit with the thoughts and agitations of the body while meditating? How do you accept what you see so that you are no longer agitated by your feelings and thoughts?

See, the saying is the practice begins when you meet that first level of resistance, meaning the push back of either mental or physical discomfort. This may mean you can't reach your toes in a forward fold or clasp your hands in a bind. Handstands and inversions seem morbidly impossible. So instead of going through with it step by step, you allow the big picture to discourage you.

Think of all the things in life that we in our highly judgmental, result-driven world shy away from just because we mentally can't see ourselves doing something. The desire is there, but logic overshadows the desire.

It's not the handstand or clasping the hands that we want to obsess over. Those will be our aims. The thing you shoot for to ensure direction as you grow. We want to fall in love with the willingness to kick up and attempt a handstand even though you're scared to death of falling on your head. We want to fall in love with not reaching our toes in a forward fold.

The lessons of yoga will shine light into every aspect of your life and give you a cool-ass yoga practice.

I'll be using the character Rory throughout this book to tell the stories that will unveil the layers that you peel back by following this method. Rory is a character created in my image, and things that have transpired in my life inspire a lot of his stories. His battles with death, purposelessness, relationships and physical pain all have one thing in common. He must learn to **T**rust, **R**eveal, **A**ccept, and **P**ractice in order to reach liberation.

Chapter 1: ME and my Soil

IF THERE IS water dripping on the floor, you search for the leak before you clean the water up. In order to understand the struggle, you must first learn the source.

It's a very tough task to find the light in certain situations, but if you train your mind to spin the narrative, you will find it easier and easier to discover the good in every situation. The way to do this is to look at your roots.

This is your foundation. Your comfort zone. The space where you identify yourself is here. This is where your fear, doubt, and judgment lives. This is also where your confidence, strength, and integrity lives.

Many people try to keep the faulty memories buried tucked deep within, creating a new image for themselves that no one can see through. Oftentimes, people use their success as a new shield. Some use their bodies and sex appeal to hide from their past battles.

Bullied kids are the adults toting guns. The current version of themselves is not being protected. There is a child inside, that they are protecting. They fear someone revealing them as weak or afraid, so they grab a weapon to look bold. They want power and respect because they lacked it as children.

These are all examples of unhealed wounds. They are the seeds planted in your soil that have yet to be nourished in a way that allows your story to blossom. If you fail to tend to the seeds in your soil, unpredictable weeds will grow at stages and points in your life when you least expect it.

The great thing is that it's never too late. You observe the seeds and nourish them. Notice I did not say you have to dig up the seeds. Our mission is not to uproot anything; our aim is simply to become aware and nourish that which comes up.

Understanding the seeds in your soil is a vital way to discover how and why you approach obstacles in life. The way you do anything is the way you do everything. Inversions are a monumental part of a yoga student's practice. It's a badge of honor to finally stick the handstand, hold the headstand, or get your butt up on a shoulder stand. It's a proud moment with good reason. However, the satisfaction that I want you to observe is not at the end. I want you to see the flowers that bloom from you just beginning. Yes, sure, the person with years of gymnastics training looks amazing as her toes point perfectly to the skies. Her backbends are pronounced in a shape straight out of the books. That person has the aesthetic but has to do more to reach her level of resistance. When I use the word resistance, I mean discomfort, a pushback from the mind and body, so to speak. That bug in your ear saying you can't accomplish something or that you aren't good enough, so don't even try it.

Resistance is what we are met with when a task seems impossible or scary, so we shy away. It's the hesitation to kick up in a handstand for fear of falling. It's the excuses that immediately come up. *I'm too old, too heavy, my knee hurts.* A flurry of doubt floats through, and you finally make the administrative decision to sit out any attempts that may lead to hurting yourself or your ego.

There is an undeniable connection between the way you approach all aspects of life. The immediate fear of getting hurt supersedes the prospect of going up. For this reason, we must look at the roots to find the answer to the question. Is it the handstand that matters, or is it the audacity to kick up without an obvious answer to what will happen?

We want to begin the mindset of falling in love with the process instead of the progress. Yes, you read this right. Fall in love with the process, not the progress. Progress is short-lived, but the process is infinite as long we continue on our path. Your yoga practice will reflect this. You will have days where certain poses are not attainable and you will have days where you can do things you never thought were possible. Highs and lows are a part of the journey; accepting this truth in your personal story is integral to your liberation.

Chapter 2: Rory's Story

This moment will forever be planted in my soil.
Will the seeds grow to be weeds or flowers?

ON SEPTEMBER 6, 2010 in the cold, air-conditioned hallways of
Beaumont Hospital, Rory was aimlessly pacing back and forth. His
large caramel hands ran across his forehead. He was fighting back
tears, but his bald head was dripping with sweat.

"Rory. I know this is tough, but you have to decide. Your mom
has been in a tremendous amount of pain. Every organ is essentially
shut down on her. The ventilator is the only thing keeping her alive."

*What is going on? Why would I have to decide? Rory thought. This
can't be happening again. God, please don't take my mama! I'm too young
to be going through this shit again. I'm 18 years old. Why are you asking
me to make the decision? WHY, GOD??!*

"I'll give you a moment alone to be with your mom, Rory."

*None of this makes any sense, how could a person be fine a week prior
just to be completely lifeless the next week? Rory thought. First my daddy,
I can't lose my momma. AHHHHHHHHHHHHHHHHHHHHH!*

When he stepped back into the room, his lifeless mom was lay-
ing with both eyes open. She was alive, but unresponsive. She was
relying solely on the ventilator. Full of emotions, Rory struggled to
digest the reality of the moment. The agony wouldn't allow tears to
fall. Just gut-wrenching screams of *why*. It was impossible to explain.

Impossible to express. Screams were the only thing that could display the emotions. Rory faced the decision to let go or hold on.

Ma…Ma…Ma…Please say something. I don't know what to do. Ma…Maaaaaa….MA!!!!!! Rory cried and moaned. *They are trying to make me let you die. Ma.. Please tell me what you'd want……*

Just as Rory was lying on his mother's side, a nurse came in to clean the various tubes inserted through his mom's nose and mouth. As the nurse pulled one tube out, a rush of blood followed. His mom's eyes grew large, and Rory screamed.

"What the fuck are you doing to her?!"

The nurse jumped back in shock.

"I'm sorry. I'll clean this up and leave her alone."

They alerted the doctor of the disturbances.

Rory's face was full of tears now.

"What is going on? Why is she bleeding from the nose and mouth? What are y'all doing?"

"Rory, your mom's organs are all shutting down at an exponential rate. This, unfortunately, is part of the process."

"What process?" he asked, crying. "Death?"

Rory sobs in distress.

The doctor nodded to confirm.

"There's not much we can do, Rory. It's going to keep getting worse the longer she's on life support."

Rory stuffed his head into the blanket at his mom's bedside, suffocating his screams. As he lifted his head up, he forgot his great aunt was in the room, sitting in a chair across from the bed. Watching with a stone face and not a tear shed.

"You may as well let her go on to the good lord," she said. "Ain't no sense in hanging onto her body. Ain't no soul in there."

Rory's aunt was his grandmother's sister. She was 87 years old and had seen many people come and go. Rooted in southern mentality, she carried her faith on her sleeve and never questioned the Lord's work. She was also the backbone to Rory's entire family tree. She said the uncomfortable without hesitation, and with her niece lying on the hospital bed, she once again was ready to say the uncomfortable.

His vision blurred by tears, Rory looked through the open eyes of his mom. She couldn't acknowledge him by sight or feel. A machine fed the breath coming through her lungs. All signs were pointing toward her life being gone already.

Just three days prior, Rory had visited her at her hospital bed. Her voice had been weak, but she'd been alert. He'd sit there with her for hours that day, with her sleeping most of the time. When she woke up briefly, Rory's mom had spoken with a weak voice, "I just want to be sure that y'all are gonna be fine. And that Deedee never ends up alone in a home."

Deedee was Rory's disabled sister. She was born the same year as Rory, just 11 months after. Irish twins, they're called. Rory was born in January and Deedee in December of the same year. Deedee was born with cerebral palsy and never learned to talk, walk or eat on her own. This was a task to which Rory's mom had given her all. Deedee was everybody's favorite, and not once had she ever had to be cared for by anyone besides Rory's mom.

Rory spoke as firm and strong as he could to give her the assurance and strength she needed.

"Ma, you don't have to worry about us anymore. We are grown, and Deedee will never be alone. We got her."

The soft "Okay, good" that followed as she closed her eyes again was the answer to the question Rory would face just three days later. She was ready to rest, but before she could, she had to let go.

With her soft, "Okay, good" in his heart, Rory made the tough decision to let her go. The nurse came in almost immediately to remove the ventilator.

"How long will it take?" he asked. "Will it be painful?"

"It all depends on the person," the nurse said in a military tone. You could tell this was just another day in the office for her. "It could take one minute or hours, but it wouldn't be any more pain than she's already experiencing."

As they unhooked her, they asked Rory if wanted to stay in the room.

Rory quickly replied, "Naw, I'm out of here."

Rory's aunt pulled up her chair and said, "Well, I'm staying here with her."

With one foot out the door, Rory stopped and turned around and sat beside his mama, too. With a face full of tears, he watched every single inhale she took. It wasn't a struggle, just an extremely deep gasp.

INHALE…

EXHALE…

INHALE…

EXHALE…

INHALE…

EXHALE…

The pause after that exhale was long.

Her chest was no longer moving. The nurse used her fingers to shut her eyes closed.

Rory screamed out one loud groan from the pit of his soul that shook the entire hospital.

"AHHHHHHHHHHHHHHHHHHHHHHHHHHHHHHHH!!!!!"

He then laid his head on her lifeless body. Eventually, the tears stopped and everything went silent. It was almost like the world had stopped.

"She's gone now," the nurse said. "Go home and get some rest."

The process was so fast and then it was over. Life happened so fast.

The ride home was silent. At 4 a.m. the dark streets had little movement. Somehow, Rory missed his turn twice before making it to the house. The ride was very symbolic of how his life would be for the next year. Dark, with Rory often lost and confused about where he was going.

MORE ON ME

One of the greatest benefits of developing a yoga and meditation practice is the internal view you gain. The practice offers a perfect opportunity for you to see everything that lies inside of you. It unfolds and uproots things that are housed in our soil for years. Things that we have either forgotten or strategically buried to protect ourselves from heartache.

Yoga is extremely humbling to even the strongest person. Just like peeling an onion, you may shed a few tears as you work through the layers. The tissues of the body houses the traumas of our past. There's scientific evidence that supports the saying, "We hold our issues in our tissues."

However, trauma is not what happened to us. It's what happens inside of us because of what happened to us. In order to release these issues, we must first acknowledge that the issues are there. There is a very common tendency to recognize only the ailments that scream for your attention.

Take a car accident, for instance. We understand the effects it can have on our bodies as we check for any breaks or contusions. We even head to the hospital to check for internal injuries or whiplash.

We typically miss the internal response the body has within the webbing of our fascia. There is a hardening that happens and most aren't able to feel it or see it. The trouble is we go years and years holding this traumatic experience without ever releasing it. This leads to a hardening of the body.

The great news is that one of the greatest ways to release trauma is through embodiment practices, such as yoga. It is very common for a student to have emotional responses during a yoga class. They are breaking through layers of trauma that have been housed for years. This is a healing experience. *Leave it all on the mat* is the phrase. Shedding sweat and tears as you release the chains from the experiences you've housed for years.

I will use the analogy of soil to help you visualize the things we house in our bodies. In the same analogy, I will use water as a reflection of everything intended to nourish our soil. As you realize what comes up, you'll learn to place yourself into fertile ground that will allow you to release and then flourish flowers wherever you stand.

Chapter 3: Water

You must water the soil, expose it to light. You must pull the weeds that threaten the growth of your flowers.

Water is essential to life. So let's look at everything that nourishes our soul as water. We want to be mindful of the foods we eat, the people we allow in our lives, and the things we say to ourselves.

ONE OF MY most impactful experiences to come from my yoga teacher training was my understanding of the impact food has on my body, mind, and emotions. Prior to the training. My family taught me to eat all the food on the plate. The mindset was to eat until I'm full. The most filling foods were those heavy in carbs, grease and sugars. We drenched vegetables in seasoning and sauces to add taste and flavor. Making the food soulfully pleasing every bite.

I can still taste it now. Monday's fried pork chops, rice and mac and cheese. Tuesday fried chicken, sweet peas and mashed potatoes. Friday was take out day, so a burger and fries from McDonalds. Saturday we would do pizza and then Sunday it was everything you could think of because we'd go to the basement at church for dinner. Soul Food to the core.

See, this is the way we ate. It was a time for family and bonding. Food was our love language. The bonding was the true soulful part of the meals. The unfortunate part is that those foods tore a hole into the core of the family. Diabetes took limbs from family members only 50 years in age. High blood pressure ensured everyone needed their meds after meals. The heart attacks rumbled through the family. Then, without a doubt, cancer stuck his toe in. There are tons of research supporting the theory that the waste we keep in our bodies can in fact turn into disease.

Through my yoga practice, I looked at the foods entirely differently. Every time I ate heavily the night before class, my stomach felt weird. Whenever I twist left or right, I could feel a log in my belly. I felt heavy overall when attempting inversions, even though I knew I was strong enough. I was seeing the impact the food I ate had on my body and would wonder how it affected the rest of my day.

The only dietary advice I will give in this book is to pay conscious attention to your body during mediation and yoga. I am not interested in giving a bunch of theories or fad diets. My only ask is that you begin by practicing with these steps in mind.

1. Avoid eating heavy meals before practice. Try to curb your appetite with nuts or lemon water.

2. Hydrate yourself before and after practice to encourage healthy recovery. It is completely normal to feel sore after yoga. Just like with any other physical activity, the body needs time to adjust. You do not need days to recover. Get back to it.

3. Pay attention to how you feel in practice the day after eating lower-vibrating foods such as processed foods, dairy, sugars, and alcohol.

4. Avoid overeating during meals. DO NOT eat yourself full. 75% of your stomach capacity is ideal.

5. Drink an 8oz cup of room temperature water before each meal.

6. Avoid eating no less than 3 before bed.

7. Walk your meal off after eating.

Being conscious of the impact foods have on your body will be more life-changing than a diet. We are creating a lifestyle, not a diet. Take on the mindset that you are learning to observe the impact certain foods have on your body. Note the way you feel as you are cleansing your body and nourish your soil. There is much more you can do, but this is good for beginners.

Confidence is everything

What you speak about yourself creates a vibration that attracts the words you say. What you speak is the water you use to nourish your soil. Words of negativity grow weeds, words of empowerment breeds flowers. Perspective is everything, so having that softening of the mind where you speak positivity is very important.

I am not tight. I am light
I am not weak. I am strength.
I am not unstable. I am able.
I am not depressed. I am impressed.
I am love.
I am well.
I am whole.
I am exactly where and who I should be.

Chapter 4: Flowers & Weeds

> We have a choice at each given moment to
> observe the flowers or the weeds.

FLOWERS ARE THE pleasant things you notice in your life. Flowers come in a myriad of shapes and colors. Like Tupac famously said, *if a rose grew from concrete, would we really care about its imperfections or would we simply applaud its courage to defy the odds stacked against it?*

Well, the flowers I speak about can grow from concrete situations. The obvious flowers will hit you in the face. These are the pleasant things like being loved, accomplishing a goal or the feeling of peace. Those are the obvious flowers, but often amid a moment, we miss the other flowers that present themselves. An example would be a car jumping the curb plowing into your home, barely missing yourself and your family who were in the backroom enjoying a movie. The shock and disappointment of the damage would be the weed, the flower in this case would be you being in the backroom instead of the front.

It is easy to become blinded by the tunnel vision created by our desire to reach goals. When I first began practicing yoga, I wanted to look like the models on social media. I obsessed over the look so much that I didn't realize that I had come pretty far on my yoga journey. I never mastered the poses, but I had gotten much further in my forward folds than before. That was a win in my eyes and shouldn't be ignored based on the comparison to anyone else.

Acknowledging the small wins along the way is important in keeping a progressive direction along your journey. The awareness to acknowledge what fuels the mindset needed to reach new heights. So when I say there is no measuring stick on success, I mean there is nothing too big or too small. Celebrate your victories and then continue on your journey. It is dangerous to obsess about goals. Chasing what isn't, instead of appreciating what is. There is a need for balance in all aspects of life. Too much chasing means you are missing life, too much celebration means life will pass you by.

It's important to note that we smell the flowers, not obsess over them. This is the power of non-attachment. Good and bad things get the same treatment.

Weeds

Like the flowers that grow, weeds are nearby, growing just as fast. The weeds aren't a person, place, food or thing. It's the unpleasant sensations we feel when dealing with people,places,food or things. Weeds can be obviously bad things, but can also be inconspicuous things that we like but turn out to be bad. I love ice cream but learned that the lethargic feeling I have after the pleasant taste is gone makes it actually a weed. I think we can all identify people we thought were pleasant but ended up displaying weeds.

Although weeds can be sparked by a person, we don't want to identify the person and play the blame game. Instead, you observe the sensations that result from interactions with the person. If they bring out flowers, smell them. If they bring on weeds, you must pull them to ensure your environment remains fertile.

Cleanse Your Environment to Create Fertile Ground

There's two types of friends: the drainers and the gainers. You want to surround yourself with the people who vibrate higher. Those that truly master seeing the fullness of the glass opposed to the empty. Friends are just as important as the mate you choose. No matter how positive you aim to be, if misery surrounds you, it is likely to pull down your vibration. Insert yourself into a room full of believers. Even if you feel odd or new to the space, insert yourself. A good yoga studio offers more than yoga. They offer a community that breeds positivity. You want to be in these types of clubs. It's necessary for your well being.

The other side of the coin is running away from aversion or things we don't like. This is equally dangerous, as we have no clue of the gift lying inside of challenges until we go through them. With so much focus on the future, it's easy to miss the beauty in the now.

There has to be a deliberate focus on finding the flowers within every situation. As you pull the weeds that do not belong. This is not always easy, but it is necessary in your journey toward liberation.

Chapter 5: The Moon

Your highest aim in life is your moon shot. This will guide you throughout your journey. This becomes your reason for getting up every day. This becomes your light in the darkest moments. This becomes your reason for moving forward. This is where you put your energy. You'll discover your purpose is here as well.

Growth is the key to happiness. With your aim in mind, every day you grow. There is no measuring stick on aims. Nothing is too large or too small to pursue. You should have an aim in everything that you do. This does not mean making goals you know are likely to be accomplished. You should set aims that meet the eye and exceed the eye.

Often, we marginalized our aims to limit the odds of failure. It's this mindset that buries dreams and kills souls. The mindset that allows us to pursue things that are not before our eyes is that of a child. Free from doubt, fear or hesitation, a child explores the possibilities of the world. With an open heart, we can tap into that world again.

Imagination of a Child Is Something Special

Imagination is the most important ingredient for growth. Knowledge is limited, but imagination encircles the world.

Logic will get you from A to B. Imagination can take you to places logic would never allow. Imagination taught us to try things that are quite scary—for instance, walking. This may sound pretty minor, but think about the bravery and determination a child must have to get up and attempt steps for the first time. Unphased by the high possibility of crashing to the floor, for a child, each step is a new opportunity to get closer to their dream of walking like everyone else.

This child-like bravery is necessary for everything we attempt for the first time, including yoga. The beginning is quite daunting, walking into a studio without a clue what is about to happen. You've heard of the benefits, but the fear of being judged seems to wash out your recollection of why you signed up for such embarrassment. I mean, it has to be shameful that an adult can't touch their toes, right? How about standing on one foot?

These are maybe some fears that people face stepping into a class for the first time, and I can tell you firsthand it feels pretty ridiculous the first time on the mat. But. What if you looked at yourself not from age but from experience level? Meaning, accept your infancy as you explore the endless possibilities of your practice. You may be older in years on earth, but you are a baby in the world of yoga. Having your aim in mind will keep you on the mat despite the discomfort you have stepping into new space. This, once again, is a mindset shift. Think about the countless things you have pursued in life, then think of the discomfort you felt first stepping in. This discomfort will lie within any aim that exceeds your current conditions. We are changing our relationship with discomfort. Next, I am going to allow Rory to share how the imagination of a child can propel us to levels that exceed the eye.

Rory's Imagination

I was 5 years old, and I can vividly recall my only friend. My best friend wasn't anyone from school or in the neighborhood. He lived in my head. My imaginary friend Bloppy. With him, anything was possible. Literally anything.

I once flew off my grandma's porch belly first after Bloppy convinced me that if Superman could fly, so could I. He encouraged me to take matters into my own hands at my grandparents' house. I had told them countless times that I was bored.

The newspaper I stuck into the flames of the stovetop was supposed to be a trick to see how fast the newspaper would burn. Well, after I tossed it into the trash can, an inferno lit up the kitchen!

I got beat down that day. Both of my grandparents whooped me, and then my mom got a piece of me when she got there. Later that night, when my dad got off of work, he bit off the last piece of my ass that remained. It felt like I was being jumped into a gang.

That was the last of my fire show displays.

Then, another time, Bloppy was the host of a wrestling match in my bedroom. I was part of the main event vs King Pillow.

It was off to a grand match. Back and forth we went. But then King Pillow latched onto my face and went to slam me on the bed. King Pillow was a dirty fighter. Somehow. My head missed the mattress and caught the wooden edge of the bed frame, blasting a hole into my forehead. Blood was all over the room. My mom lost her shit.

"What the fuck did you do?!" she screamed as she sped me to the hospital. "OH MY GOD! OH MY GOD! Keep the towel on your head. What the fuck were you doing?!"

Fourteen stitches later, the nurses laughed as I told them about the wrestling match. My mom was completely over it. She didn't find me or Bloppy funny. I could see it on her face.

On the way home, she told me I need to get rid of this imaginary friend if he was going to keep getting me messed up. My dad was way more direct. He looked me right in the face and told me. "The shit is fake, man. You're too damn old for imaginary friends, anyway."

I realized they were right. I was almost 8 years old, still talking to an imaginary friend. It was time for me to grow up!

Imagination vs Logic

That was the beginning of Rory being thrust into the limited world of logic. The world's blueprint for success limits the creativity of the soul. It's the first layer of entrapment, typically. We are to go to school, get good grades. They have studies that show how well kids should do at every level. The same curriculum applies to every single kid regardless of their background, circumstances, and unique interests. I am not saying this isn't necessary for the development of a child, but as I continue explaining, pay attention to the box that is being created.

By the time you are 9 or 10 years old, you would have likely been introduced to extracurricular activities like sports, dance, robotics, art, etc. Those first ten years of life, I like to say they are molding you, and based on what you excel at, that becomes your niche.

Run track if you are fast, play basketball if you have some height. Play football if you are a big kid. Girls, they teach you to put your dress on and stop being so sassy so that people will like you. You are good at flips, so cheer is for you, and don't even think twice about picking up your brother's football.

The world of doing what has already been done. Even more damning is only doing what you excel at instead of what your heart desires. If you move outside this box, judgment and shame will whip you back into it. Yes, logic is the most dangerous tool used to control the imagination.

I remember playing basketball in the backyard every single day. I would watch Penny Hardaway on TV, then go back outside to practice the moves I saw him doing. You couldn't tell me I wasn't going to the NBA. Was I any good? Not really, but I had a lot of fun playing.

Well, until my uncle told me I needed to focus on football because basketball only has five spots on the court, so my odds of making a football team were greater. A logical suggestion, shaping a box around my desire to hoop.

It's not always done in spite; most often it comes from a place of love. The people closest to us often fear witnessing the heartache. The history of black people has an extra layer of logic for good reason. Society forced entire generations to protect themselves and their families. Some imagined better for themselves and their family and would risk it all to pursue the impossible. Others took on the mindset of protecting their current state so that they didn't lose or harm what they already had.

This goes back to the soil and moon analogy. The person who is uncomfortable in their soil has no trouble deciding whether to pursue their aim. They have little to lose. It's the person who has found comfort in their current situation who runs the highest risk of becoming fixated and allowing life to pass them by.

Mindsets get passed down from generation to generation until someone is bold enough to break through the chains of comfort and into the world of endless possibility. These are the chains Kanye West speaks about in his "rants." If you set aside your judgment and the splurge of words that often make people miss the initial point, you will hear something similar to what I am saying now: Success and failure are both relative. It's when we allow society to decide what is or isn't desirable that's when the box forms. There is no good or bad. There just is. If we can see that everything that is, is and everything that will be, will be, then we can experience life without the limits of our mind and others' expectations.

There are countless families that still, to this day, limit what their kids can do or say in order to protect them from shame or harm. A softened stance on what is logical and what isn't can only release this handcuff.

The Webster dictionary defines logic as "a proper or reasonable way of thinking about something" but does not include the unique views of the person. This strips away the emotion and intention behind an act and instead focuses on the act itself. So when I say logical, I mean this extremely loosely as a way of saying "inside-the-box" thinkers. Those who look at life from a measure of good or bad outcomes. They miss the lessons because they are looking through the lens of the past instead of seeing the truth in the now.

It's very easy to take on the logical mindset. It's comforting because most times you'll have others who see things the same way. You'll have more supporters as you set aside your dreams for something more logical. The exact opposite of a logical mindset will require you to tap into the unthinkable side of your brain to see things like a kid again. Kicking up for a handstand because you want to fly instead of shying away so that you don't break your neck.

What Rory's parents didn't realize was that Bloppy was playing a huge role in his development. The fearless curiosity of life requires the ability to balance falling and flying. Actually, I'll let Bloppy share his side.

Bloppy's Perspective

They try to label me the bad guy, but I'm actually his best friend. The only loyal friend that is around for the good, bad and ugly. I watched him fight back his tears to avoid being called a punk. I sat with him as he buried his emotions because y'all know the saying, "Big boys don't cry."

Every time Rory felt anything, they whipped him back into the box that society created. Now I may get things wrong sometimes. I may even cause a little pain, but I never try to keep him from being alive. Who wants to go through life sharing someone else's story? How many people can say they've set an entire kitchen ablaze without burning the house down?

Then, that wrestling match was epic. Rory was having the time of his life. I don't know what made him turn away from the bed and face plant into the floor.

Yeah, Rory may not acknowledge me as much as he used to, but I'll always be around. I'm the voice in his head. It's me that screams "You can do anything!" I'm also the voice that screams "Stop, don't do it." It's up to Rory to decide which to listen to. He was good at deciding until he began pretending I didn't exist. Now he thinks he is the voice in his head.

His parents were ready for me to disappear. However, if they'd looked a little closer, they would have seen the many success stories that come from exploration because of me.

Inspiration Comes from All Places

Inspiration comes in all shapes and forms. It's not limited to those doing better than you. Someone that is not in the field can inspire you. We gain inspiration from the results a person has as well as their process.

I remember close to my 30th birthday; I began looking at my life and the lives of others a lot differently than I had previously. The non-attachment aspect of yoga was something that I had gotten deeper into. I was seeing the beauty of people just trying to live out their desires.

I was never a fan of LeBron James until he left Cleveland for Miami in a move he deemed best for his life at that moment. The pressure that came with that big move was much greater than even he could have expected. I watched the seasons in Miami, where he was still a tremendous star and won multiple championships. Still, I noticed a hesitation in him when taking certain shots, and in his post-game interviews, he almost seemed like he was giving an excuse for his play. The next season, however, when he went back to Cleveland, I watched an interview where he vowed that he no longer felt the pressure of winning or chasing the ghost of MJ. Instead, he said he was enjoying the game, and he vowed to celebrate every chance he got. He had this awakening where he realized his career wouldn't last forever, and that you can miss a lot of great things by being obsessed with only one bar for success.

That season, I noticed him taking shots in games, and when he missed, his post-game response was simple: "I missed the shot."

That's a simple way of saying, *Shit didn't go as I hoped, but I'll see y'all tomorrow to try again.* This was inspiring to me, even from a career so different from my own. But in my head I decided there's shit that doesn't go as planned every day, but I'm going to take my shot, anyway. Miss or not. Rory had an experience similar to this as a kid. One that I'm sure we can all relate to.

Take the Training Wheels Off and Experience Life

Rory saw a kid riding his bike down the street. He was going so fast. Rory tried to keep up with him, but couldn't. The boy noticed Rory behind him and screamed, "YOU ARE GONNA HAVE TO TAKE THOSE TRAINING WHEELS OFF IF YOU WANT TO KEEP UP WITH ME!" as he laughed.

The wheels that were protecting Rory from falling were keeping him from going fast.

He asked his mom, and she told him to ask his dad. His dad said *Okay* as he blew him off five days in a row. They were hoping Rory would forget and stop asking.

One day, as Rory sat on the porch, his neighbor pulled up. He was always working on something: Cars, cutting the grass or just fixing stuff. He must have sensed Rory's desire to get the training wheels off.

"You want me to take those training wheels off for you, Ro?"

He was the only person who called Rory "Ro." Rory hated it, but didn't care, as long as his neighbor was going to pop the extra wheels off for him.

"YES!! I've been waiting all week to get them off!"

"Go ask your mom if it's okay, and I gotcha."

Rory ran into the house with excitement.

"Ma! Mr. Oakfield said he would take the training wheels off for me!"

She looked at Rory and said, "No! Your ass is gonna fall and bust your head again!"

With tears in his eyes, Rory replied, "Ma. No, I'm not. I promise I won't fall."

They went back and forth for 30 minutes. At that point, Rory had snot running down his face from crying and begging.

"Ma, please….please, ma! I'm the only person on the block with training wheels still. MAAAAAAAAA PLEASSSSSSSE!!!!"

Then finally, she broke her hard stance.

"Okay, I don't give a damn. Let him take them off, but they are not going back on."

Rory didn't even let her get the rest of her words out before he rushed back out with a smile and a snotty face. He looked at Mr. Oakfield.

"She said yes!"

But Mr. Oakfield must have heard the back and forth between Rory and his mother, so now he was hesitating.

"You sure, Ro?"

With a screechy voice, Rory said, "Yes, I'm sure!"

Like two peas in a pod, Rory and Bloppy worked on riding this bike. It was like *The Little Engine That Could.* Rory was the train conductor on the bike, and Bloopy was the engine inside his head, pushing him to keep trying: *I think I can... I think I can.... I think I can....*

Rory stayed out there for hours. He fell countless times, and with each fall, he learned a little more.

Don't look left, don't look right, don't look up and definitely don't look down. Look straight ahead and keep pedaling.

Suddenly Rory was moving. He was doing it. His body was stiff as a board. But who cared? He had it!

Rory screamed at the top of his lungs.

"MA!!! MA!!!! I got it! I got it!!!"

She yelled back immediately.

"I see you, boy! You go, boy!"

At the time of Rory learning to ride his bike, he wasn't aware that this same approach would guide him through every obstacle he'd face in the future.

There were a few monumental mindset shifts that happened because of Rory setting his aim of riding without training wheels. His aim was the target, but the stars that appeared along the way created a lasting impact.

1. **No matter where the desire comes from, if the heart yearns for it, we should act on it.**

2. **Be persistent. Accept "NO" as resistance, not rejection.**

3. **You will not always have support. Although Rory's mom loved him, she didn't want to imagine the joy of him riding because she was blinded by the fear of him falling again.**

4. **Do not waver. Once you set your aim like a hawk in the trees, zero in.**

5. Lose your attachment to the results. Warned that the training wheels wouldn't be placed back on, and presented with the possibility of falling again, Rory still stayed the course.

6. Patience is the surest route toward mastery. Rory cut away any thoughts of failure or success and focused solely on one pedal at a time.

Don't look left. Don't look right. Look straight ahead. Fears planted inside

Rory's mom had been watching the entire time. With each fall, she'd cringe, but the most important thing she watched was every time he got up. Often the fears that are planted in the soil of kids are based on their parents' fears.

They fear two basic things: losing what they have, and it happening again. This fear keeps them from being the greatest version of themselves and teaches them to limit the child that they are raising. All rooted in fear. People fear losing what they have earned or, in Rory's mom's case, what god has given her in a son. People also fear the pain that they experienced previously happening again. So instead of experiencing the fruits of life, they set back in the safety zone. No flying or falling. They sit still.

You can look deeply into every time you are hesitant, from the smallest thing to the biggest, and you will see one of these two fears in there.

What Bloppy offers is the stark contrast to this limited mindset. He offers encouragement to see. Bloppy doesn't know the result of anything, and that's not his job. He is simply the voice of reason.

Just a smidgen of inspiration often sparks the desires we have in life. The random guy riding down the street inspired Rory. The imaginary voice in Rory's head was his only ally as he reached for his aim of riding with no training wheels.

This was a monumental point in his life but also in his mom's life. She no longer felt like she needed to protect him. She could trust that no matter how many times he fell, he'd get right back up.

Just like a child learning to ride a bike, you must be steadfast with your aim. Your aim is straight ahead, and you should not waver with your focus.

The Small Wins Lead to Big Mindsets

Don't look left. Don't look right. Look straight ahead and fix your focus on your aim. This concept is another universal truth of life. It's imperative that we have our vision fixated on an aim to keep us from being distracted by external factors that may be in the room. In yoga, this is called a drishti in Sanskrit, but in English it's called a gaze point. Gaze points are used throughout the duration of your practice to center your focus. It's known as the gazeless gaze simply because we look past the tip of our nose, but not necessarily at anything. The view is still inside. This empowers your practice and keeps you in the moment.

Your yoga practice is very symbolic of the way you approach your life. Often, the limits we have within our minds are consistent. It's for this reason it is of great importance that you let go of your attachment to results in order to experience the process of yoga unfolding before you.

This means you are not forcing yourself into crazy shapes or images that you've decided in your head that you must master. That is the ego taking over your practice, and this is often how injury happens. Part of the practice is learning to balance the art of pursuing more and surrendering to the now. The posters you see on charts or in videos are often images of master yogis with extreme levels of flexibility. There is absolutely nothing wrong with that, and I'm not for shaming the person who can place their head between their legs, or the person who can't. These figures create enough aim in a posture so that the common yogi has something to work toward. The aims that we set are inspirations, not destinations. Although we may reach the destination, and we may in fact want to, we still understand there is plenty of fruit along the journey. You see where you want to be, but you understand that the glory comes from the things you observe along the way. We will call the poses the aim and the soil your current state. The stars will be the things you realize in yourself along the journey in pursuit of the aims. Aims are important in all aspects of life, so it's important that you have multiple aims. One in every category of your life: social, health, financial and mental.

Inspirational Trigger

Inspirational triggers go much deeper than the success of someone's efforts. Their lifestyle can also inspire you. I remember telling a client of mine about my interest in yoga. She painted a picture of a lifestyle her neighbor lived that intrigued me instantly.

"Oh my neighbor, he's a yoga big shot. The guy lives a glorious life. He goes to work for an hour or two in the morning, then before noon he's back at home in his big, beautiful house. The guy seems like he doesn't have a worry in the world."

Her hard Asian accent was clear enough for me to draw the picture in my head. I could see myself going to work for a couple of hours doing massages instead of sitting in the spa working seven hours. Maybe I could have clients all over the world, doing massages wherever I went. My imagination was churning simply off the brief lifestyle picture that she'd painted.

I wondered if I could take my current situation doing massages and make it into a lifestyle where I was only working a few hours and enjoying life the rest of my day.

I had no cemented plan of action, but the concept of living more while working less seemed lovely.

My aim was the lifestyle, not the person. I began noticing people all times of the day casually going about their business. They didn't seem in a rush to get anywhere or stressed by anything. I wanted to live that lifestyle, but I was afraid of losing the security the spa gave me. I needed to tap into a mindset that I had dumped many, many years ago. I needed to enter a "but-less"world. A place where "but" didn't exist. The mindset of "anything is possible." The only way this but-less world could exist is if I allowed myself to notice the beauty in the journey.

Chapter 6: STARS

THE QUOTE "SHOOT for the moon and fall among the stars" suggests that you will fall. I like to say, *Shoot for the moon and see the stars along the way.*

It's common for people to only see two things. The beginning and the end. This is the win-or-lose mindset. This keeps us trapped by results. You must learn to embrace the process, there are loads of beauty and wins along the way.

If the soil is the beginning and the moon is the end. Then the stars are the journey. The stars are things you notice in pursuit of your aims. It's the things that we typically miss because we are so fixated on our desires. Although we must remain focused on the aim, we do not want to be blinded by it. There is so much life happening before our eyes that we don't fully comprehend to be a star at the moment.

Throughout your yoga journey, it is important for you to take the scenic route as you pursue your aims. Every posture will present a new opportunity to see inside. There will be so many things that expose itself along the way. Old injuries, trauma, pain and aging joints and muscles. You don't want to enter the practice by jetting to a destination. Hoping to master a pose. What we want is to master the acceptance of what you see inside of you throughout each pose. No matter where you begin if you can begin observing everything within your practice. You'll soon discover your purpose somewhere along the way, as everything in your life will soon become a star. Trust what you see and all is coming.

Set Your Aim but Expect It to Move

Often, we mistake our purpose in life to be a graspable thing. We believe that with tremendous efforts, we will reach our highest aim. We believe that the promised land will fulfill our lives. In reality, our purpose is not a place, it is a state of mind.

The aim is not to be obtained, it's to be pursued. The aims give direction. By letting go of our obsession with victory, we realize that our lives are aligned with our purpose. What you may view as the highest aim may become the foundation for something greater, or the direction that leads to your purpose. Enjoy the scenery, and life will not be as daunting. It's only one step at a time. One day at a time. One breath at a time.

The first and most important act of gratitude should begin with yourself. I appreciate myself now. I speak positivity in my life as I pursue higher aims. Life may take me downstream and back upstream, but there is always a sight and life to see. If you obsess with the aim, you will strip yourself of the joys of life. Pursue your aim and feed yourself the fuel for a forever satisfying life. This is how we use the practice to liberate ourselves both on and off the mat.

Amid any actions, there are two things that determine feelings. One is sensation and the other is breath. Yet people rarely focus on those two determining factors..

Think about times where you were in a pleasant mood. You can probably imagine the smile on your face and maybe even laughter. If you looked deeper, you would also notice the ease of your breath and the calmness of your heart. You are free from restraints. You want to bottle this feeling up and keep it forever. In a perfect world, we would all be full of pleasant sensations.

What if I told you there is a way to view all sensations as pleasant, and you don't have to hopelessly try to bottle up any moment?

Yes, realize the pleasant smell of the roses while they are before you. Live in the now and trust that whatever comes next is to serve you as well.

On the same coin, distress is the other side. These are the times where you have felt immense anger. Often during anger, we black out and almost lose control of the moment and begin reacting to what comes up. You are then fighting a sensation instead of accepting it.

Trying to battle your frustrations with more anger is like standing in the center of a lake amid a windy day. Trying to stop the crashing waves is completely impossible.

What is possible, however, is for you to observe the waters as they are. You'll notice there's beauty within the crashing of the waves, and as the storm passes, there is equal beauty within the stillness of the waters.

If you take the observer approach with yourself, you will see beauty within the frustrating moments and the pleasant ones. You practice watching the changes in mood instead of letting it dictate who you are. Not that you won't have moments of anger, sadness or fear. This is the beginning of you practicing the mindset that frees you from the suffering of feelings.

Those who aren't conscious of these sensations will continue to be victims of the feeling. You have a choice to observe the waves of sensation as a moment, or to bottle all your frustrations and give them a damning name or explanation that weighs on you: *Moody, grumpy, or I'm having a bad day.*

We want to take the approach of breaking down what you feel into sensations instead of balling it into a mood. The person who recognizes that they are angry is no longer identified as angry. They instantly become the observer of anger. This is a much safer position to be in.

Am I really so angry that I want to cause so much strain on my body? Most would likely say no. Immediately, anger loses its control over you. Your decisions become your own. You rationalize the moment instead of becoming a byproduct of the tornado created by the human tendency to wrap thoughts and feelings into a singular word to describe a moment: *Anger, Frustration, Joy and Happiness.* The words of the dictionary have been misrepresenting feelings for an entirety. We take back our power by not identifying ourselves with any label. Allowing ourselves to just simply be.

This is an arduous task, yet obtainable with practice. The interesting thing about the body is it knows no difference between good stress and bad stressors. So we can develop your ability to observe uncomfortable situations without an associated reaction within your yoga practice. Yes, the trials of a yoga class can generate great turbulence in the mind. You find yourself in a battle with your thoughts and feelings. If you aren't conscious, you just may mistake a moment for a bad day. *I'm tight today!* Or maybe you keep tipping to the side in balancing poses and think, *I have a terrible balance.*

These are labels that do not help at the moment. They harm the mindset as you think back for past signs of confirmation that you are in fact unstable.

One of the more hated is boat pose. The sensations that come along with boat pose mimic those that I used to explain anger. I can't tell you how many classes I have taught where the students are either gritting their teeth in agony, or holding their breath waiting for it to be over. Some decide to throw on the stone face and fight the boat back with bicycle curls. The boat pose is the undefeated champ; however, it has beat the best of us down in the battle of who's gonna tap out first.

However, the physical is only one angle that I want you to view the posture. Instead of grinding your teeth and screaming, you are to observe the breath and the sensations that come up in the body. Be the observer without labeling yourself. For example, *I feel discomfort in my lower back, but that does not make me weak. I feel my legs trembling, but that does not stop me.* You learn to signal to the body that changes in sensation are natural parts of life. There will be pleasant and unpleasant moments in your yoga practice. I beg you not to fall in love with the enjoyable moments because they are not lasting, and I beg you not to run from the inopportune moments because they aren't lasting either. They are both unavoidable truths of life. We will undoubtedly experience good and bad moments in life. Learn to observe both the same way you can accept the sun shining and the moon rising. Both play a role in this wonderful, interconnected universe we live in.

Nothing Last Forever

Rory's parents' deaths were a direct example of impermanence. Meaning nothing good or bad lasts forever. Death is the most gruesome form of impermanence, but a definitive part of our life cycle. Realizing this does not end the pain, but it can relieve you of the suffering. It is not the emotion itself that causes the disturbance. It is the array of thoughts that come along with it.

Let's take a plane ride, for instance. The anxiety of riding 40,000 feet into the sky can be terrifying. Even before you leave the ground, the thoughts of what could happen begin. Once in the air, the first rumble of turbulence causes a flurry of thoughts to run through your mind, causing you to wonder again. *What if?*

It's at this moment where you should begin to observe what *is*. We can break the feelings of discomfort into digestible chunks of what *is*.

I can feel the sweat in my hands, the pound of my heart, the shallow breath as if the thought of the plane going down is reality.

When you catch a glimpse of the flight attendants' calm face, you place things into perspective and begin to realize that the reality of what you feel is turbulence, you calm down. In order to reach the destination, you will experience spurts of choppy air. *What if you looked for the calm you seek in a flight attendant in yourself?*

This is a basic concept of life. In order to reach your destination, you accept that there will be moments of turbulence that you must breathe through and realize what *is* instead of what *isn't*. The turbulent mind eventually fades. It is my belief that watching my parents die gave me a gift of understanding that nothing lasts forever. By accepting impermanence, you begin living life instead of trying to avoid death. Pain is a fact of life, suffering is an option.

Rory is going to take you through his journey of life after pain.

Part 2: The T.R.A.P.

Chapter 7: Trust, TODAY

THERE MUST BE a sense of surrender in everything we do. An ability to let go. Once you have learned to surrender to the moment you are prepared to embrace that which lies inside.

Life down the dark path of the unknown is scary. The great thing is we no longer have dark alleys to walk down. We have flashlights and maps on our phones that can guide us to the doorsteps of any destination. No longer do we rely on instinct to get home.

The eery path that we are afraid of is the unknown. Before we take the next step, we want to see what's in front of us. We want a complete layout of the map that shows at a high probability we will reach a desirable place. We do this in careers, relationships and health. Show me what's in front of me or what's in store for me, and I will go.

Unfortunately, life will often thrust you into the dark path of the unknown. Rory did not know what the next steps in life were. Much of his decision making went through his mom first. What was he to do? How was he going to navigate this foreign territory?

Life happens for you not against you. SAUNA MAN.

The days after his mom's death, Rory received several messages of support. Mostly kind words and stories of how to cope with loss. Rory received welcoming and unwelcome gifts from friends of his mom.

He received three bibles, four bottles of Hennessy and a couple of pre-rolled blunts. Some believe, prayer is the answer, while others believe drinking and smoking away the sorrows is the key. Rory wasn't interested in any of it. His greatest source of peace came isolated at the gym.

The gym had become a place Rory used as an outlet. Slinging weights and running miles gave him the release of anger that was lying in the pit of his gut. With every weight pushed, there was a release of frustration. With every mile ran, he was separating himself from the sorrows of reality.

He was trying to escape from his thoughts, but just as soon as he stopped running the memories would come back. The isolated runs would be the place where the mind would get the best of him. He saw blood in his mom's mouth as they removed the tubes. The questions, the thoughts and the visions never stopped.

She will never get to see me married. Never hold her grandbaby. Never get a chance to see me become who I am going to be. Why would this happen to me?! How is this even fair?!

It was an episode that would play much too often and would bring him to tears all the time. He couldn't run fast nor far enough to outpace the rabbit mind of misery while ailing from the loss of his mother.

One particular day at the gym, Rory thought about a future without his mom. In the middle of bench-pressing, his lips quivered with tears, filling up to the brim of his eyelids. The only way to save himself from embarrassment was to pick himself up and spend the rest of the time in the sauna.

It's no way I'm letting anyone see me crying in this fucking gym, he thought. *Damn, I miss my mama.*

Rory grabbed the towel to wipe his face clean, then placed the snotty towel over his head and rushed to the sauna where he could zone out without a lot of traffic. He could be alone with his thoughts, sweat and tears.

About five minutes in—as Rory was sweating, and feeling a lot better—the door opened. Massive feet stepped in. Rory didn't bother to look up.

Oh god, someone is coming in. Please don't talk to me. I don't feel like having any sauna tal, Rory thought.

Oh god, someone is coming in. Please don't talk to me. I don't feel like having any sauna talk.

The big-footed person flopped onto a seat across from him. His deep vibrating voice asked, "You good, bro? I saw you struggling on the bench up there."

Wow, this guy probably thinks I was crying in pain because of some weights, Rory thought.

"Oh yeah, I'm good. Thanks. I wasn't crying up there."

Fuck. Did I just tell him I wasn't crying before he even brought it up?

"Okay, well if you ever meet someone who does, tell them not to fight their emotions. Life is much easier this way. If you fight your feelings, they'll control you. Accept them, they'll free you."

Gandhi is gonna force me to talk to him, I see.

"Yeah, man, some stuff should private, though. I have a lot on my mind, but like I said, I wasn't crying." Rory insisted.

"Nah, that's actually where we get it wrong, bruh. You should be able to embrace your emotions wherever you are."

"What does it prove, though? Let's say I sit in the middle of the gym crying like a baby. People would think I'm soft, suicidal or just plain crazy."

Sauna Man shakes his head.

"Labels have been screwing us for generations. We can't do one thing or another because of the labels that people have placed on us. These are the chains that keep people trapped in place. It's why people fear being seen. This is part of the reason I told you to accept your emotions."

"Yeah, I hear you, but as soon as you show your emotions people take your kindness for a weakness. They tease you, manipulate you or even worse, they pity you. I don't want anyone's pity, and I don't want anybody thinking I'm a punk."

"All that's understandable. My question for you is have you ever determined what you want? All I hear you saying is what you don't want."

"It's not always clear what I want or even who I am. All I know is that it sucks terribly to lose people you love. The two people I've been living my entire life to impress are gone. So I have no clue."

"Well, the best place to begin is with who you are not. I can tell you confidently that you are not who they said you are."

"Who are *they*?" Rory replied.

"Society, young bruh. The fears you have of being called a punk or being taken advantage of are not new. It's the wicked way the world has taught men to believe. Mask everything because we are the display of strength. Express anything and you are dubbed weak. Those are labels that hang us, and we have the power to cut the rope."

Chapter 8: Titles

Titles, labels, and names kill the essence of who we organically strive to be.

WHEN RORY WAS a kid, his parents would drop him off at his uncle's house in Atlanta for a month during the summers. This was his dad's brother and also where his grandparents lived. He didn't care, he still hated being away from his mama. One day she called to check on him. Hearing her voice over the phone broke him down every time.

"Ma, I want to come home." Rory burst into tears.

"I know, but you'll be okay, you only have a couple weeks left. Can you be a big boy for two more weeks?" his mom replied.

"Yes." Rory sniffled.

"Good,

that's my boy. I love you and I'll be there to get you in two w,eeks. You can start counting now. And try to stop crying, Rory."

"Okay. I love you, too. Bye."

Immediately after Rory hung up the phone, before he could wipe the tears off his face, his cousins walked by to greet him.

"Awww, Sissy misses his mommy."

Next Rory's uncle walked in the room.

"Uh oh, here comes the crocodile tears again."

They all laughed as Rory sat alone. At 9 years old, the shame of showing his emotions taught him to never cry in front of anyone again.

Titles kill the essence of who we are and who we are to become.

Titles—The Silent Killer SUCCESS

The losses we have are shattering. They bring on pain that most would crumble from. We all want to win and will do anything to capture the title. The title of best, enough, better than everyone else. It covers us in superiority as we boast at those beneath us. My crown is large, and yours is not. I could not imagine a life where I'd have to sit the crown down.

A life where I'd have to come down from my high horse or lord forbid I'm knocked from it. I've always chased the crown and always knew that in due time I'd reach it. I started so young I have plenty of time. My parents made sure I was good at everything. *Do your best and be the best at everything you do.* Your life will be a success.

Atlas I reached the crown and stared at the face of success but inside I felt useless. There's nothing up here. It's weird. Everyone can see me and they are waiting for a mistake. Was it a mistake coming up here? Where do I go? It's nowhere to go but down. Wait what's going on? Are they kicking the bottom? Are they trying to knock me down? I'm afraid but I can't let them see me weak. I've been faking my smile for so long.

They are going to call me crazy like Lauren Hill when she reached the peak. They are going to call me odd like Kanye West when he finally cracked. I don't know what to do. Why the fuck was I so determined to get up here? Why didn't anyone place a caution sign next to this crown? Why didn't people warn me about the empty crown? What will I do now?

Maybe I'll share my fears and depression. That's what I'll do. I'll tell everyone below that it's not so cool at the top. It's actually pretty depressing up here.

Hey everyone, it's not what you think! I'm really pretty empty up here!

"Shut up and enjoy your pretty life. Enjoy your great job,big house, family and beautiful smile. We don't want to hear that shit. "

No really,it's all a facade. It looks good but nothing on the inside. Why are y'all so mad and heartless?

Never mind, I'll be fine, hand me my crown and mask. I mean my smile.

This smile I wear is becoming worn out. I wish someone taught me how to lose the same way they encouraged me to always win. You are not your success.

Titles—The Silent Killer FAILURE

Each title that we wear creates comfort, no longer lost in the world of identifiable you are happy to call yourself something. There is a dark path to becoming, and the fear is that you will never reach the light.

I look left and right. There's a light right there so I'll just settle here. I've been on this dark path far too long to not known for anything.

There's so many people here it's comforting to no longer be alone. Where am I?

"This is the comfort zone, it's a ton of us chilling here. Take off your shoes and you can stay as long as you want. There's a fireplace over there. Our only ask is that you throw your dreams there so that the fire stays ablaze and keeps us comfortable."

Wait, burn my dreams? I don't want to do that.

"I'm sorry you may be in the wrong place then. You can head back out into the dark whenever you are ready."

It's hard to see anything walking out there.

"One step at a time in the dark you must step. The becoming is not a destination it is an endless journey where often the only light you have is the light that burns inside of you."

You will see so much and if you are aware, you realize that step by step is the only thing that matters. There will be turmoil and there will be joy. Your job on this journey is to recognize these obstacles for what they are but to never confuse it with being who you are. You are not a failure.

Titles—The Silent Killer MISERY.

This dark path of the unknown is tricky. You may know your direction and have your faith but life has other plans. Its brings on unexpected pain that makes you question why.

My mom would be so proud of this journey I am on, if only she was here. Damn I can't believe my mom is not here to see this. Why am I even going anywhere? It's pointless. I have no reason.

"Hello! Hello! Look this way over to your right. Come over here we can help you. Our name is SORROW. We have a place for you to lay."

"Hey no don't listen to them. Come this way you should be ANGRY. No one deserves to lose a parent, come over here! Let's tear some shit up! You deserve to rage and vent."

"Hey! You're in a dark place just come over here. I got everything that makes you feel good. Your favorite drink, some good food and pretty girls."

I just need a break, that's all I just need to feel good. You think I can chill here for a minute with the girls and food. I'll have one drink as well. What do you call this zone by the way?

"Welcome, it's called the cravings zone. We have everything your soul craves to make you happy. But beware we are only temporary and there are side effects to being here. It may set you back on your journey, maybe even change your life."

You are not your MISERY.

You are not your sorrows.

Titles Do Not Define People

The overwhelming part of titles is that they restrict the person's ability to be anything else. Titles have a way of blinding the individual of what is because they are completely convinced that they have already become. They have found a zone to be known by. This is very dangerous as we know life changes unexpectedly, and our desires do as well. Often people are afraid of uncomfortable feelings so they are quick to label themselves with a title to protect themselves. I realize serious diagnosis like cancer, diabetes, anxiety and depression need to be diagnosed and treated properly. The question I have is are you treating the anxiety or the person. You are not your ailments.

Trapped

At the moment Rory wasn't receiving much advice from folks who offered it in his time of grief, but the words of the sauna man were penetrating his consciousness. Rory wanted to hear more.

"What do you mean by people being trapped?"

"Well, people are afraid to expose themselves to the world, so instead of doing what the heart desires, they stay still and put on a mask. Some people wear professional masks like PhD, MD, or Attorney. Others wear the mask of baller, playboy, pretty, or funny. Abused people embrace the title of victim. People stay in relationships just to maintain the title of having someone. Bullies put on tough guy masks because they are afraid of being seen as weak. Some people put on temporary masks to hide their emotions as they come up, and others wear them permanently."

"You can't really blame a person for putting a mask on to protect themselves. It's our instinct. People are mean, they take advantage of your weaknesses as soon as you open up." Rory looked up for agreement.

"It's not about blame. The real question is, are you living a life of action or reaction? If you are deciding based on the actions of others, then in fact you are a reactor, meaning you have allowed yourself to be controlled by emotion. This is a very dangerous mindset because at any moment someone can influence you to do something you will regret."

Rory rubbed his head.

"Nah, I'm not bad like that. I just know certain things not to do in front of people or say because it will cause them to say something or think of me differently."

"My friend, I know you are thinking this is not a tremendous deal but if you consider the trickle effect, you'd understand my point. You're bottling up emotions, both good and bad, that are meant to be freed. That's a recipe for a volcanic explosion."

"Explosion? I'm not like that." Rory laughed.

"None of us are like that until we are." the Sauna Man said. "Sometimes you'll feel like crying, so cry. Some times you'll be mad, so be mad. Some point you'll be happy. Go 'head and be happy."

The Sauna Man gathered his things to leave.

"The main thing is to let yourself feel all the feels, but don't let your feelings at the moment dictate your entire day. Have sad, mad and happy moments as a natural part of an adventurous day that ultimately tells your unique story. This does not mean your day or your life is ruined. These are fleeting emotions that should be acknowledged and let free. Share your story, and your days will always be free from the weight of life."

"Wait what do you mean when you say share my story? Like are you saying talk to a therapist or something?"

"I mean talk to anyone who wants to listen. Your story is not limited to the words that come from your mouth. I saw you on your phone when I came in here. You can share your story on social media. The way you express yourself. Facing your fear of shedding tears is a way of telling your story. It's a powerful way, actually. Be bold, my dude. I'll catch you next time."

Just like that, he left. What the Sauna Man was trying to get Rory to see was that there are two options in life: acceptance or suffering. Suffering comes when you are tied to the teetering emotions of pleasure and pain. We all have that friend that believes the world is against them. They blame every misfortune on an issue that they have yet to let go of. Acceptance is when you embrace both as flowing truths of life. Acceptance allows moments to come and go regardless of what sensations they brought along with it. Suffering happens when your happiness depends on the existence of pleasure and the avoidance of pain. Neither is lasting, neither is unavoidable.

The Sauna Man's words stuck with Rory.

Moments not days, be adventurous and share your story.

You can run through the fire of life and live to tell about your wounds. Or die hiding behind the smoke, leaving someone else to tell your story.

Chapter 9: Funeral

THE DAY OF his mom's funeral, Rory walked in without a tear in his eye.

I felt in my stomach like I should release, but the tears had dried up. I couldn't cry. Her body didn't look like her. I had seen her body go through the process of life to death. This was only a shell of my mama.

As the funeral went on, the pastor asked for people to share kind words. Person by person, Rory watched as family and friends tearfully shared stories of how they knew his mother.

I could hear them speaking, but I couldn't register the words they were saying. It was like I had entered an underwater twilight zone. I could only think about what I would say. I hadn't even committed to saying anything, but the way my heart was beating, I could tell I needed to say something.

By the time the last person spoke, Rory had built up the courage to stand to his feet.

My stomach turning into knots, I was questioning if I needed to speak or run to the bathroom to poop. Who was I kidding? My gut was telling me to get up and say something about my mama.

Rory sternly stood up as if he was being called to join the US Army. His three sisters sat in the front row. He was taking the first steps to display strength for his family.

Still unsure what I should say I began doing exactly what the sweaty Sauna Man advised:

"Run through the fire and tell the story of the wounds. Don't run through the fire, someone else will tell how you died from the smoke."

Rory had already been through the fire of watching his mom die but he risked dying from hiding from the story. I do not mean dying to be taken literally, although perhaps the long-term effect of bottling stress will lead to death. *That which you keep inside will kill you, that which you let out will free you.*

Rory went on to the stage to thank everyone who paid respect. Maintaining his composure to display strength and saying all the things a man should say at a time like this.

"My mom was a great mom but she would not want to see us crying. She would want her life celebrated." Rory displayed a smile to assure everyone that it was ok to dry their tears.

As Rory scanned the room, he accidentally made eye contact with one of his mom's closest cousins from Kentucky. He was always so country-strong and the image of a man's man, but today his face was covered in tears. His lips quivering. Eyes red.

That eye contact was enough to break through the shield Rory was hiding behind. Rory began crying uncontrollably, breaking the firm soldier's display that he'd planned. A groan that mimicked the sound from the hospital came from the pit of his soul. He paused to recoup.

Suddenly, the memory of his mother's final breath began flowing out like a river breaking through the dam, the detailed account of his mom's last days, all the way to her final breath. Rory spoke with a broken voice. He was no longer speaking to empower his family; he was now speaking to free himself. Half of the story came out, while the other half remained choked in his throat.

"I was there every day witnessing death before my eyes with my dad.

I thought that was the most difficult thing I'd ever have to face. I had no clue less than a year later I would stare at my mom in the same light.

Cancer left me staring in her motionless eyes as she lay on the hospital bed. Waiting on me to decide. To hold on or to let go."

They are trying to make me let you die. Ma.. Please tell me what you'd want....

I begged for an answer. I buried my head into her chest. Deep down I knew her exact wishes, but I wanted her to say it. One of the last days she could talk. Her voice was so weak at this point almost like she was whispering. She expressed her desire:

"Rory I just want to make sure your sister Deedee will be taken care of. The rest of y'all can fend for yourself but she needs her family to take care of her, not a group home."

"I promised her then, as long as I'm alive. Deedee will never spend a second in a group home. I watched as she took her last breaths.... one at a time.... her chest went up and down.... Deepest breaths I had ever seen.... I imagined death being a struggle, but this wasn't a struggle. She had no more fight in her. It was her final exhale that felt like the biggest inhale of my life.... I was inhaling life as she was exhaling life.... that last breath was her last gift to me. It was her time to go and my time to live."

It wasn't the powerful delivery that Rory would have hoped for, and the message didn't roll out like he'd wanted. His words were filled with sobbing pain. But as he sat down, he thought about the ultimate words that he'd said.

"It was her time to let go and my time to live." Rory had been alive but only in the image and footsteps that his parents set in front of him. This is a scary time, because he would realize he has no directions. He was taking on guardianship of his disabled sister Deedee and would soon realize that there are no directions manual on her and none on life.

Chapter 10: Be Authentic

THE ONLY WAY toward healing is to be completely and undeniably authentic. Often there are no words that can explain how we are feeling. That is ok and you should not drive yourself crazy trying to say how you feel. Vulnerability and being authentic sometimes sounds like a sob instead of words. The way you express and release has to be genuine to you. This may mean journal your thoughts onto paper before sharing it with the world. Some may choose to dance as a way of expression. The laughter and tears shed when sharing should not leave out any detail. There is no right or wrong to let out that which lies inside of you. The only thing that matters is that you get it out.

The words that Rory shared hardly mattered, it was his willingness to be brave, bold and vulnerable despite the overwhelming levels of nerves. It was the first step of freeing himself by telling his authentic story.

There is no rule book for authenticity. The vivid details that Rory shared were exactly what had to be done to begin the healing process. You cannot fluff and buff your way towards liberation. You must be able to reveal, accept and relinquish your truth.

His mom's cousin's pain triggered Rory, it revealed his own. This led him to sharing a perspective of his mom's final breath that gave him peace at the moment.

This didn't mean that the feelings of sorrow would magically disappear forever, this just meant that Rory had decided to not allow his sorrows to define him in that moment. He vowed to use his account of death as a reason to live out his life fully.

Live Your Life

In the months following the funeral, life hit a weird intersection. The phone calls and text messages to see how he was doing stopped. People were back to normal while Rory was still ailing. He couldn't decide what he wanted to do with his life. After making the bold statement of living his life to the fullest at the funeral, he faced the scary reality of actually doing it.

Rory had no kids or a girlfriend. His only company at the houde was his sister DeeDee, who he'd promised his mom he would take care of. That would prove to be a expectede anticipated as well.

Deedee had a severe case of cerebral palsy. She couldn't walk, talk or eat on her own. She completely depended on Rory's mom for everything. It was the moments where he didn't have the answers to his sisters need where he would struggle the most. Task that he was now responsible for included bathing her, doing her hair, taking her to doctors' appointments.

Brushing her teeth. How on earth did she get her to keep her mouth open? Rory would often cry in frustration.

He felt so electric and free after being vulnerable in front of the people at the funeral. Although it was an emotional take on the life of his mom, it also was a liberating one.But now in the midst But now amid easier to lay in sorrow. ie in misery.

My mama is gone forever. This is ridiculous. Why should I take care of anyone? I don't have kids. And when I do, Who will I call when I need help? Who will my future kids call grandma? Who will tell stories about how I was as a kid? This is horrible.

Confused and out of ideas, Rory headed back to the gym hoping to run into the Sauna Man again.

Sauna Man Strikes Again

That morning Rory walked around the gym pretending to lift weights, trying to make out the face of the guy but he couldn't recall anything besides…

Those big-ass feet! Where the hell are you, big-foot Sauna Man?

After about 20 minutes of watching people pump iron, he headed down to check the sauna. Sure enough, the big-ass feet were there. With a big smile, Sauna Man's voice vibrated out.

"What's up, my man?! I had been thinking about you."

Sweat dripped from his coarse gray beard. He took the towel off his head, revealing his cleanly shaved bald head.

Somewhat hesitant to reveal the truth, Rory smiled.

"Man, everything has been good. Just managing the best I can."

"That's all we can do is our best."

Rory sat down in the corner away from him so that he didn't feel obligated to talk, but deep down he was dying for Sauna Man to ask him about the funeral.

"How did the funeral go—and everything after?" Sauna Man asked.

Whew! Thank you for asking!

"The funeral was one of the toughest and most liberating moments in my life," Rory said. "I took your advice, and I shared my story. I literally spilled my heart out in front of everyone. I felt empowered in the moment but that feeling didn't last. My days have been very sad. I keep finding myself in sorrow. Almost like I'm allowing life to defeat me. My thoughts drown me, and I can't think of another way of getting out of the funk. It's not like I can speak at a funeral every day."

The Sauna Man was no longer smiling.

"You had a mouthful there. The story you shared at the funeral was the key to your enlightenment, not liberation. You felt liberation at the moment because you began shining your light by sharing your story. What you discovered is your life purpose."

Rory looked up, slightly confused.

"My life's purpose is to tell people about my mom dying?"

"That and more. Your story in life can be a weight in your belly weighing you down in sorrow, or it can be a light illuminating the world with inspiration. We are the most alive when we share our experiences with others. Both the good and the bad."

"So who should I be telling my story to? And how will I know what story to tell?"

Sauna Man flashed a powerful grin now.

"That's the magic of life. We don't always have the answers, but if you allow life to flow, the answers will present itself. I can't tell you what story to tell only you know that."

Rory was more confused than ever, as the sweaty Sauna Man stood up to leave.

"I gotta head to work now, but I'm usually here during the week around this time. Keep me posted on how things are going. One last thing: The universe is a stage where you don't have to wait for an audience to be heard."

As he exited the sauna, Rory looked at the clock and realized he had to be to work in an hour himself. He was a Massage Therapist at a spa Downtown Detroit. It was a cool job when he was in a pleasant state of mind. When he was in a bad head space, it was torture to spend hours in silence as he provided services to clients. Thoughts would shower his head this day as he continued to think about what the Sauna Man was telling him this time.

Chapter 11: REVEAL

THE WORKDAY WAS pretty normal. Typically Rory would see a variety of different clients. Some would talk through sessions and some remained quiet. Today was a talkative day.

Rory's last client for the day was a regular, Ms. Hoo with two O's is what she went by. Rory respected her opinion and enjoyed having conversations with her even though her English was difficult to understand. Her slight frame and big smile was always a warm sight for Rory. She would always tip before the session and bow her head in thanks to show appreciation.

Rory was happy to have a conversation with someone who wasn't aware of his mom passing. Instead, she was interested in hearing about his football boys. Go figure, an older Asian lady interested in hearing about youth football. Gotta love the diversity of Detroit.

Rory volunteered coaching the little league football team that he'd played for as a kid. He coached the 9- and 10-year-olds and always had a good story to tell about them.

"So what's new with my boys? Are they winning? Any funny stories for me?"

"They are doing pretty good. The season is just about over now."

Rory didn't have the courage to tell her he hadn't been able to coach all season because of his mom passing.

"After the hot summer months' training and conditioning for the season, the boys always get catty. Managing their emotions, making sure their grades are good. That's the biggest task," he said. He tried his best

to make up a believable story so that he wouldn't have to explain why he hadn't been out there.

"They really blessed those boys to have a cool-headed coach like you to help them navigate life."

"Yeah, and I love watching their maturation. They come to us as babies but leave as young men by season's end. The wins and losses never matter to me."

Ms. Hoo had opened the Pandora's box to Rory's passion. He lit up talking about them the rest of the session.

Later that evening, Rory thought more about the conversation. Not so much what they'd talked about, but more about how he'd felt as they spoke. He'd felt electric, alive. It was a feeling he hadn't felt since the moment on stage at his mom's funeral. He believed that maybe his purpose was out on the field with the kids.

The next day, he gave one coach on the team a call. He had been running the show with a couple other volunteers during Rory's break. Loud and crazy Coach P screamed through the phone.

"Coach Ro! I'm glad you called me, man. I was about to knock down your door if I didn't hear from you soon. I heard your mom passed."

After offering his condolences, true to form, Coach P let Rory know exactly how missed he was.

"Man, I've been waiting for you to get back out here to help me with these badass kids! I think they are tired of me, too, they keep asking when Coach Ro is coming back. I told them don't worry, he's gonna be back and when he is, I'll be disappearing for two months my damn self!"

They both broke out into laughter. Coach P had a way of using his humor to engage the kids, and they loved him to pieces for it. Parents from other teams would stick around just to hear his pregame speech.

For most people in their early 20s, the last thing they'd want to spend their summers doing is working, let alone volunteer work, but these boys were Rory's soft spot.

These kids from the heart of Detroit came from backgrounds completely out of their control. They often found themselves on the team to stay out of trouble or to gain discipline in their lives.

We were not just coaches but also mentors in charge of being a positive example, a light, so to speak, Rory *could see a little of himself in all of them. Just ten years earlier, he was out on that same field sweating and learning so much from the wisdom of his coaches.*

Tenacity, perseverance was etched on the jerseys. The words that inspired Rory were now being channeled from his voice to their ears.

The team greeted Rory the first day walking out to the field the same as usual. He appreciated the normalcy. One boy saw him and screamed.

"YESSSSS!! Coach Ro is back!!"

With a face full of joy, Rory gave him five and asked how he was doing.

"Good, just been here working out. I heard your mom died. I'm sorry to hear that." His face went from serious to a smirk quickly. "You want to race? I got faster while you were gone."

The pure sincerity in the voice of this 10-year-old as he offered condolences, followed by an immediate challenge to race, gave Rory the instant confirmation that he was in fact exactly where he was supposed to be.

"After practice we can race, but for now give me two laps."

As the boy darted off to run his laps, Rory watched his steps in appreciation.

This is exactly what I needed. I had been feeling so sorry for myself, that I had forgotten the things I enjoyed in life. Rory thought.

It became pretty clear that what actually lit him up was being out on the field. That light would only last two more weeks, however, as the season was already at its end. Rory would once again have to discover his purpose. The next months were a rollercoaster. Temporary highs followed by startling lows. The balancing act of living a normal life and caring for Deedee was getting the best of him. Rory needed a break.

Chapter 12: Run Through the Fire and Tell the Story of the Burns

ONE DAY BEFORE his birthday, Rory sat alone by a pool in South Beach, 1300 miles away from the frigid winter of Detroit. This would be his first birthday since the passing of his mom. Isolation had become his approach to dealing with reality. He didn't have the desire to celebrate with anyone without her midnight voicemails starting off his day.

"Happy Birthday to you! Happy Birthday to you! Happy Birthday Dear Rory! Happy Birthday to you! Answer your phone, Niggah! I know you ain't sleep. Call me back. Love you."

Rory's mama displayed a crazy mix of motherly compassion and "friend from the street". They had an unexplainable connection they'd shared. They would talk about god, girls, school, work or just good ole drama from a show on TV.

Things didn't move Rory the way they did when he was younger. He used to anticipate Thanksgiving dinner even more than Christmas. Rory would hound his mom about having the food ready before the football games came on.

"MA! When is the food gonna be ready?! It's almost 12 o'clock!"

"Shut up! The food will be ready whenever it's ready. You ain't got no damn in-house chef."

Rory would laugh every time he got a crazy response.

Christmas and New Year's Day were all Rory's favorite times of the year. His mom cooked enormous meals, and all the sports came on then. But with his mom no longer around to harass during the holidays, they no longer excited him. Birthdays were not a big thing anymore either. Rory had a hole in the center of his heart that any other voice on earth couldn't fill. He had become distant from family and any friends that reminded him of his mom. It was his way of coping.

Christmas and New Year's Day were all Rory's favorite times of the year. His mom cooked enormous meals, and all the sports came on then. But with his mom no longer around to harass during the holidays, they no longer excited him. Birthdays were not a big thing anymore either. Rory had a hole in the center of his heart that any other voice on earth. He had become distant from family and any friends that reminded him of his mom. It was his way of coping.

Christmas and New Year's Day were all Rory's favorite times of the year. His mom cooked enormous meals, and all the sports came on then. But with his mom no longer around to harass during the holidays, they no longer excited him. Birthdays were not a big thing anymore either. Rory had a hole in the center of his belly that couldn't be filled by any other voice on earth. He had become distant from family and any friends that reminded him of his mom. It was his way of coping.

Christmas and New Year's Day were all Rory's favorite times of the year. His mom cooked big meals, and all the sports came on then. But with his mom no longer around to harass during the holidays, they no longer excited him. Birthdays were not a big thing anymore either. Rory had a hole in the center of his belly that couldn't be filled by any other voice on earth. He had become distant from family and any friends that reminded him of his mom. It was his way of coping.

The trip to Miami was purposely planned to take him thousands of miles away from family. He left to roam around South Beach the next three days alone.

Go with the Flow South Beach

The next day, the glare of the rising sun woke Rory. He stood out on the balcony and watched the waves from the ocean crashing as the sun reflected far away. It was so hypnotizing, the waves and breeze. He wanted to get closer. So he threw on some shorts and a t-shirt and strolled down to catch the sun as it rose. This was a perfect time and a peaceful place to begin his meditation practice.

As I approached the shore, I realized my phone was not in my pocket, sucks I can't get a picture. This sight is too good to miss, forget the phone.

Rory took his slides off and sank his toes into the warm sand. They hadn't come to rake yet. Between his toes he could feel the debris from the previous day. Rory was focused on making the best of the moment.

The seaweed and bottle caps annoyed the hell out of me, but I wasn't about to let that ruin my moment. I got closer to the ocean. I found a clear patch of sand and sat there.

I listened to the sound of waves crashing, the seagulls chirping, I felt the wind against my skin.

One inhale after another, Rory's eyes closed. He was drifting into this space that he hadn't been familiar with. It was a space of no concern or wondering. He was in a domain where he was happy to just be.

I recall reading about this place called pure bliss in a magazine while on the plane. I had never experienced it myself. This had to be it.

Inhale the good…

Exhale the bad…

Rory had long given up hope it was possible for him to feel this peaceful. The serene setting and the circumstances gave him the nudge just be present. *I wanted to be with me. I wasn't concerned with where I needed to be because I didn't have any place to be. I wasn't worried about what I was going to do because I had no plans. Life is good. What was I thinking?*

Enemies of Meditation

> If you avoid going through the fire, you will die from the smoke.

At this moment, Rory sat without a care in the world. This went on for over an hour. Motionless bliss is what it felt like.

He drifted from a seated position to suddenly lying on his back; the sun beaming on his head as he snatched his t-shirt off, baring his chest. He took the shirt and placed it over his face to guard against the sun that had gotten too hot. He was submitting to the moment.

How cool would it be to always have this perfect setting? What if I lived off the ocean instead of cold-ass Detroit? My life would be so perfect.

Just as Rory sat with the bliss of Florida, he suddenly could hear the voice of a child laughing.

"Grandma, come on! Mommy is catching up. We have to beat her. Come on!"

"I'm coming, big head boy! You are too fast for me with those short legs." A woman's voice replied.

Rory's eyes opened up to match a face with the voice that sounds so familiar. A voice pure to his heart.

I knew it was a black mama. I could feel my mama. Rory thought as the boy ran in circles excited to reach the ocean. His grandma smiled as she took her time walking in the uneven sand. Rory had yet to see the mom they were running from, but he immediately began analyzing their moment.

She has to be 75 years old if not older. Her legs swollen, and she's overweight. She has to be diabetic or have high blood pressure. Fuck, probably both. How is she alive but my mama dies at 52? How is that even fair?

This had become normal for Rory. He would quickly scan anyone that reminded him of his mom no one deserved to live if his mom couldn't.

"You better not get too close to that water. If it washes you away, I'm not coming to get you." The grandma warned the young boy.

That was totally something my mama would have said. This is so fucked up. My mama never even had the chance to see me have a kid. Get married. Accomplish anything. This sucks so bad.

Rory's thoughts about the past and the future often drove him into dark holes of depression. He knew it was unhealthy, but he couldn't find a place that didn't trigger him. Even on the sandy beach of bliss, misery crept in. Rory did what he did all too often. He got up and walked away from his thoughts. He enjoyed the blissful moments as he sat in meditation, but he missed the great opportunity of sitting through the discomfort. You can avoid the fire but yet still die from the smoke. If Rory was to find peace, he needed to sit through the recurring pain of his mother's death.

Meditation and its Aim

There is a huge misconception of meditation being a practice where you relax. You inhale all the good of the moment and you exhale all the bad. If only it were this easy. Being aware of what you feel, think and hear as you sit is a part of the practice. The aim is not to control your environment; the aim is to realize your environment. With awareness comes acceptance. With acceptance comes peace. The thoughts lose their control of you as you no longer flee from the bad and no longer cling to the good. You allow life to flow, understanding change is a part of life.

As you see Rory found himself in a pretty ideal scenario. Perfect weather and no responsibilities, yet still he was disturbed by the child playing with his grandmother. Most would find a moment like that heart-warming, for Rory this was a trigger that he has yet to notice. The true essence of the practice begins when you realize the agitators and sit with them until they no longer agitate you. Rory missed an opportunity to sit with his agitator, he became frustrated and left. He still has much to learn. You cannot outrun the turbulence of the mind. Just like a plane ascending through the sky you have to sit through the bumpy air to reach new heights.

As you see Rory found himself in a pretty ideal scenario. Perfect weather and no responsibilities, yet still he was disturbed by the child playing with his grandmother. Most would find a moment like that heart-warming, for Rory this was a trigger that he has yet to notice. The true essence of the practice begins when you realize the agitators and sit with them until they no longer agitate you. Rory missed an opportunity to sit with his agitator,he became frustrated and left. He still has much to learn. You cannot outrun the turbulence of the mind. Just like a plane ascending through the sky you have to sit through the bumpy air to reach new heights.

As you see Rory found himself in a pretty ideal scenario. Perfect weather and no responsibilities, yet still he was disturbed by the child playing with his grandmother. Most would find a moment like that heart-warming, for Rory this was a trigger that he has yet to notice. The true essence of the practice begins when you realize the agitators and sit with them until they no longer agitate you.Rory missed an opportunity to sit with his agitator,he became frustrated and left. He still has much to learn. You cannot outrun the turbulence of the mind. Just like a plane ascending through the sky you have to sit through the bumpy air to reach new heights.

As you see Rory found himself in a pretty ideal scenario. Perfect weather and no responsibilities, yet still he was disturbed by the child playing with his grandmother. Most would find a moment like that heart-warming, for Rory this was a trigger that he has yet to notice. The true essence of the practice begins when you become aware of those agitators and sit with them until they no longer agitate you. Rory missed an opportunity to sit with his agitator,he became frustrated and left. He still has much to learn. You cannot outrun the turbulence of the mind. Just like a plane ascending through the sky you have to sit through the bumpy air to reach new heights.

As you see Rory found himself in a pretty ideal scenario. Perfect weather and no responsibilities, yet still he was disturbed by the child playing with his grandmother. Most would find a moment like that heart-warming, for Rory this was a trigger that he has yet to become aware of.The true essence of the practice begins when you become aware of those agitators and sit with them until they no longer agitate you.Rory missed an opportunity to sit with his agitator,he became frustrated and left. He still has much to learn. You cannot outrun the turbulence of the mind. Just like a plane ascending through the sky you have to sit through the bumpy air to reach new heights.

As you see Rory found himself in a pretty ideal scenario. Perfect weather and no responsibilities, yet still he was disturbed by the child playing with his grandmother. Most would find a moment like that heart warming,for Rory this was a trigger that he has yet to become aware of.The true essence of the practice begins when you become aware of those agitators and sit with them until they no longer agitate you.Rory missed an opportunity to sit with his agitator,he became frustrated and left. He still has much to learn. You cannot outrun the turbulence of the mind. Just like a plane ascending through the sky you have to sit through the bumpy air to reach new heights.

As you see Rory found himself in a pretty ideal scenario. Perfect weather and no responsibilities, yet still he was disturbed by the child playing with his mother.Most would find a moment like that heart warming,for Rory this was a trigger that he has yet to become aware of.The true essence of the practice begins when you become aware of those agitators and sit with them until they no longer agitate you. Rory missed an opportunity to sit with his agitator,he became frustrated and left. He still has much to learn. You cannot outrun the turbulence of the mind. Just like a plane ascending through the sky you have to sit through the bumpy air to reach new heights.

As you see Rory found himself in a pretty ideal scenario. Perfect weather and no responsibilities, yet still he was disturb by the child playing with his mother.Most would find a moment like that heart warming,for Rory this was a trigger that he has yet to become aware of.The true essence of the practice begins when you become aware of those agitators and sit with them until they no longer agitate you. Rory missed an opportunity to sit with his agitator,he became frustrated and left. He still has much to learn. You cannot outrun the turbulence of the mind. Just like a plane ascending through the sky you have to sit through the bumpy air to reach new heights.

You Can Run but You Can't Hide

Rory stormed off the beach. His mind was about to wander into a worthless, pitiful tangent, the rumble of his stomach grabbed his attention. It was time to eat. Instead of going back to grab his phone, he began walking toward food. He had no restaurants in mind as he walked aimlessly down busy Ocean Drive. He was kinda hoping to get lost, something to take up the time of the day.

His headphones were at the hotel, so he had no music to accompany him. People were just making their way out for the day. Rory walked swiftly, trying to wash out the thoughts of his mom. He hoped a little workout would bring back the pleasant feeling he had prior to his sunbathing being interrupted. The elements were so vibrant today. The palm trees waving as the morning breeze flows through the city, sun completely out, grass being cut, the banging of new construction. Rory could hear it all.

He noticed a lady walking swiftly with a yoga mat, then saw a guy with one too. *Hmmm must be a studio somewhere around.*

He took a few more steps, and on the corner was a building with two doors open as if they were trying to air the place out.

I wasn't really interested in taking a yoga class. Still, I wanted to take a peek.

As he poked his head in the door, a lean, olive-skinned, dark-haired hair lady at the desk caught him peeking. Rigorously, she waved her hand, motioning Rory to come in.

Fuck. I knew I shouldn't have looked in.

"Are you interested in taking a class?" she asked.

Immediately Rory thought, *Hmmm not really but I'm sure you're going to suggest that I should.*

"Oh, no, I just saw people walking with mats and wanted to check it out."

"Well, I'm glad I caught you. You would have missed the best parts of the studio trying to check it out from way back there."

This lady is so damn jolly. I bet it's the ocean vibes. I need to get my ass out of Detroit more often. I'd be the same way living in paradise.

She graciously explained every offering the studio offered. Gave Rory a tour of the space and even let him peek into a class that was in session.

"Shhhh. They're in practice but they don't mind."

It was completely quiet. No music or teacher leading the class. It was 30-40 people squeezed in this tiny room, mat to mat, breathing and sweating.

Rory looked at her. She could tell he wanted answers.

Why isn't the teacher calling out the poses? How do they know what to do? Why are they breathing like this?

"This is Mysore Style Ashtanga Yoga. You come in and begin your practice no matter what time you get here. It's self practice, no comparison to anyone in the room or anything like that. You simply go through the poses of ashtanga, exploring your limits."

This differed completely from what I thought yoga would look like. I imagined an old lady with her mat laid out in the front of the room telling people to breathe peace as they touched their toes.

It was the exact opposite. To Rory's amazement, the class was filled with shirtless fit guys dripping in sweat, mixed with beautifully toned women rocking nothing but sports bras and tiny shorts.

Sheez! I may need to give yoga a shot. I popped in yoga once or twice at my gym to get a good stretch before hopping on the treadmill. It was nothing like this. This was different, much different. It was beautiful. It was like a beautiful dance of breath and movement.

"This is so cool. Do the teachers ever tell them what to do?"

"The teachers are there to help you get deeper into poses or to assist you if you cannot remember a pose. The most important part is to allow yourself to go with the flow. Have you ever done this before?" she stared into Rory's eyes.

"I mean, I've done yoga a few times but not like this. It's usually more structured. It was a teacher at the front of the class telling us what to do and showing us how to do it."

She smiled.

"Oh, well, you'll be fine. Going with the flow doesn't mean you lack structure. Going with the flow means you are okay with however you show up on the mat. You learn to trust what you feel in your body and honor it. You become your greatest teacher as within every twist, forward fold and balances pose lies a story being held in your muscles in tissues. Yoga teaches you to reveal those stories and release your attachment to what comes up. You should come back and take a class before your trip ends."

Rory left with a handful of pamphlets detailing the studio and the teachers. The back of the pamphlet read "Go with the Flow" in big bold letters just above the class schedule. The style of yoga they were doing intrigued Rory.

Chapter 13: Morning Bitch

RORY CARRIED ON his search for a breakfast spot. Just three streets up, he could see a pink awning with a massive flamingo in front of it. As he got closer, he could hear loud music. Rap music, to be exact.

What the hell? Is it a club? It's not even 10 a.m. yet.

As he got closer, he could see people eating, so he continued to the door. Just as he stepped in, a girl about five feet tall greeted him.

"Good morning, BITCH!"

"Huh?!"

"I said, welcome to GOOD MORNING'S BITCH!"

Rory, totally confused, laughed it off.

"Is this a breakfast spot? I wanted to eat."

She laughed. "Of course we have food for you. Let me get someone to seat you."

As Rory sat down, he scanned the place. The people were laughing, eating and some even drinking. They had a live DJ playing all types of music.

Wow, this bad boy is jumping early. I like this!

The server approached his table.

"Morning, bitch!" she said.

"What's up BITCH?!" Rory said.

Without a smile, the server replied, "Never call a woman a bitch! The place is called GOOD MORNING BITCH. This isn't a free pass to call people bitches."

Oh fuck.

"I'm sorry, you're absolutely right. This was a way of joking around. I'm really sorry." Rory's face full of embarrassment.

The server burst out laughing.

"I'm just kidding with you, man. I'll be your bitch for the morning. The girl at the front told me you were tight in the butt so I figured I'd loosen you up a bit."

Oh, my god. What's wrong with these people? Rory thought.

"I'm not tight in the butt."

Rory pulled his seat up closer to the table as he chuckled.

"Okay, well I'm the grandma around here. The OG of the gang. You call me grandma, OG or Queen B. Just don't call me *bitch* again and I'll let you keep those pretty teeth of yours."

What in the fuck is happening?

"I'm definitely not calling you the B word anymore. So OG it is."

"Okay, I'll take that! Don't mind me either. I like to have fun with people. It keeps me young."

The server smiled at Rory with her gold side tooth shining and glasses hanging off the tip of her nose. Her apron tied around her waist, and her hair pulled back into a silver gray bun. Her eyebrows were drawn on with an arch that made her look excited no matter what she was saying.

I wonder how old she is. Gotta be in her 60s. Why the hell is she working somewhere like this?

"Well, I'm gonna let you decide on some food." The OG server walks away.

The menu was just as funny as everything else. One side was all your typical breakfast food, and then on the other was vegan options, smoothies and green eats. At the top of the menu it read, "Enjoy every bite but don't bite my BITCH."

Each bite of the multigrain triple berry pancakes covered in whipped cream was like a taste of heaven on Rory's taste buds. The home fries and turkey bacon went down together. He took breaks in between bites to embrace the scenery. The loud music gave off a really cool vibe. Rory didn't feel so bad being out to eat alone, either. There were several people doing the same. Dining alone. He couldn't help but reflect.

I wish we had places like this in Detroit. Somewhere where the vibes are good and you don't feel weird being yourself.

There were people of all races and ages enjoying the music. It was rap music, specifically trap music.

If I ever had a place, I would bang loud music just like this. It takes everything up a notch. Rap creates a full vibe and everyone loves it. I don't know why more places don't do this.

"That's a lot of sugar on your plate, buddy. You know our people gotta watch our sugar."

I looked up as the OG server who brought me the meal was now telling me I should watch what I was eating. Unbelievable.

"I know, ma'am."

"What you eat truly affects the way your day flows. Heavy foods cause inflammation in your body that is worse than smoking a cigarette. I don't know why I feel inclined to tell you all this. You look like a healthy guy and you want to keep it that way."

She had a point but Rory couldn't help but to analyze. He had become a pro at noticing all the things wrong with anyone older than his mom. He looked at her belly hanging over the tightly tied apron around her waist.

"Yeah, you don't want to be like me. Diabetes, high blood pressure and cholesterol. I bet your mama has some of that going on with her, don't she?"

"She did. She had all three as well."

"I'm sorry, sweetie. You said she did? She passed away? You're so young."

"Yes, she died a year ago. It's fine."

I didn't enjoy elaborating on the details. It typically came with a pity party that I was not in the mood for.

"I'm so sorry to hear this. I knew there was a reason my heart asked me to talk to you. My mom passed away when I was just 21 years old," she said. "I'm gonna let you enjoy your breakfast, but keep this in mind. Pay close attention to how your body and mood react to certain foods you eat. I'm no dietitian or anything special, I'm just an old conscious lady who's done a whole lotta living in my 91 years on earth. I've seen a lot of my friends who lived pretty decent lives die because of the foods they eat."

Nourishment vs Craving

The OG server was completely right. Entire generations have been washed out by one or all three of the triple-headed monsters of diabetes, high blood pressure and high cholesterol. The way they taught us to eat was the recipe to ensure we needed care. The strategic placement of liquor stores and Coney Islands. The soul food my grandpa cooked was washed down by his famous sweet tea. It was the same thing that took his leg as the poison of sugar invaded his body. It's a drug that's taken so many beautiful souls.

Cravings

It is common for us to mistake the purpose of eating. We have been forced to watch commercials, ads, stores and restaurants geared toward our cravings. They encourage us to eat the foods that cause addiction. These foods contain artificial sugars that make us want more.

We feed it to our precious bodies, mistaking satisfaction for nourishment. The fact is, the body is not designed to break down the sticky residue of artificial sugars we place in our bodies, or the fatty grease we place in our bodies. The loads of salt placed in the very foods we eat mask the actual product, creating a salty palate for us to become accustomed to.

The egregious amounts of food digested each meal puts a strain on the entire digestive system. Instead of the body gaining the nutrients of your meal to spread to the parts of the body, they force the digestive system to work in overdrive to break down the food you have dropped in your belly, leaving you to feel heavy and lethargic.

Nourishment Over Cravings

It has sucked a vast majority of the population into the pigeonhole of satisfying a craving when hungry. The commercials brainwash us from as young as one-years-old. The cereals contain sugars that are more addictive than any drugs on earth. They use cartoon characters to grab our attention, and they dub the breakfast, "A great way to start your day!"

I remember in the 5th grade we had the MEAP Test. This was the most important test of the year because it would determine your placement for middle school. They told us to get some sleep the night before and to make sure we ate a big breakfast. Then once we got there, right at the table were 30 boxes full of… DONUTS! We were stoked to be loaded up with sugar and milk. That ten-minute sugar rush was the bomb. I could never understand why I got so sluggish midway through the test.

Well, the body does exactly what it is supposed to do. Eating sugar creates a surge of the feel-good brain chemicals dopamine and serotonin. We get the same effect from the other white powder: cocaine. And just like a drug, your body crashes after the initial high. You become addicted to the taste, so every time you eat it you want to eat more. No one would knowingly do this to themselves or their children. My sole purpose is to bring awareness to what you may have ignored previously.

Chapter 14: Selfless Acts of Gratitude

Random acts of gratitude are rewarding in so many ways, but the most direct is the vibration you give off to the universe, which is sure to come back to you.

AFTER FINISHING HIS breakfast, Rory was still sitting in the same spot, hanging onto the moment. He was swirling the last drop of water around in his cup when he noticed a lady struggling at the hotel across the street from where he was eating. She was having an extremely hard time getting a baby stroller off the shuttle bus. She had an infant in one arm and a diaper bag, luggage and stroller in another hand. Rory hopped up to offer a hand.

"You have a ton of stuff here. You got it?"

In shock, the lady replied, "Oh, well, yeah, can you grab this. And hold this, I'll come back and grab this from you." She threw her entire load of luggage in Rory's arms.

"You must be moving to South Beach."

She laughed.

"Nah, I have to be prepared, though. Babies require a lot of stuff."

"Oh, okay, I was joking anyway. I'll help you carry this stuff into the lobby." Rory laid her things on the floor, then proceeded out the door.

"Wait, you 're just gonna leave? Where are you rushing off to and what's your name?"

"I'm kinda just going with the flow today. I don't have any plans. And my name is Rory."

Straight and direct, she replied, "Okay, well, chill until I finish checking in."

This lady had a commanding way about her. She was short in build, attractive in her own unique way. The slight build, caramel skin and a short haircut that was giving Toni Braxton vibes. Rory was open to any company he could get.

After she checked in, she came back over and explained that she also was in town for a couple days just to escape the cold winter and grab some sun. She was from Flint, Michigan which was roughly an hour from Detroit. She had no plans besides chilling with her baby. They exchanged numbers and parted so that she could finish checking into her hotel room.

Karmic Energy

Throughout the day, Rory continued to roam around. He found his way to an area of the beach that was full of life. The local vendors had set up their unique shops.

In the center of the local business shops was a small stage. There was an old guy with a darker complexion standing in the center with his music banging. His voice was howling through the speakers as he entertained and sang to people who were mostly ignoring him. He had no one's attention besides Rory's.

The old man's voice wasn't the most pleasant, and the suit he was wearing was way too hot for performing on South Beach. He danced and moved end to end on the small boxed stage as if he had a full crowd to entertain. It wasn't the performance that was intriguing, however. It was the constant smile that drew Rory's attention.

He watched the old skinny man dance and sing while playing his guitar. Some people walked by dropping tips and some just recorded him. He didn't look homeless, but people figured it was the only reason this man would be up there.

He was on cloud nine, and there were no signs of him coming down. Rory copped a squat to listen. The old man winked at Rory as he propped his feet up on the chair across from him. This boosted the Old Mans confidence as he tried for a spin and dip that didn't work out too well. He hit the floor, and not a soul checked to see if he was okay.

He helped himself up.

"Whelp I think it's time for a break, these old legs are tired."

He stepped off the stage, grabbed some water and came over to his only fan.

"I hope you enjoyed the show. That fall at the end was part of the act," he laughed.

"Yeah, man, I enjoyed watching you do your thing. Very entertaining. Do you do this often?"

"I've been doing it two or three times a week for the last five years."

"Really? You just come out here and sing? What are you doing it for?"

"Yes sir, I love it. It's my passion. I've always wanted to be an entertainer as a kid but my dad would never let me pursue it. He would tell me it's no money in it and I needed to focus on an actual job. My mom told me it was nice but agreed with my dad. She thought I should focus on school or getting a job. Well, I did exactly what they said to do. I was miserable, though, man. After law school, I became a corporate attorney. For 20 years, I did it. I had been working toward goals but never my passion. I had a house, dog, wife and kids. But nothing that lit me up like getting on this stage does."

"So, you're telling me you left your family and job to do this? To follow your passion?"

"Hell nah, man. I still have my wife, and my kids are grown now. Five years ago, I retired from being an attorney. I didn't dump everything, I just knew I was missing something. That something was the curiosity I had as a child. About a month after my first grandson was born, they diagnosed me with a rare blood disease. The doctor told me I only had a short while to live. He said if you ever had any desires in life, you should probably work towards them now."

"Wow. I'm sorry to hear that. So this was the thing you did?"

"Not immediately. Over the first couple weeks I lay in misery just like a person who'd just received their death letters would. I lay on my back day after day in a funk because my greatest desire required impossible energy or just wasn't logical for an ill person. The same doctor would call to check on how I was doing.

He'd ask if I were living out my desires yet? I told him I couldn't build up the energy, nor did I have the resources to live my burning desire. I hoped to perform on a big stage. I'll never forget his words that followed. He said,

You have a burn in your belly that needs to come out, you shouldn't save or store it hoping for a perfect place to reveal. The audience that lies in front of you is perfect enough. The gift is being able to live out your desire, not the measure of what you put out. Do not half-ass it, go full-out no matter who is in attendance. You are doing this for you, not for a reward or result. Begin now."

"I remember it like yesterday singing my song. I would sing it softly to myself, no guitar, just my voice. I was singing to keep myself busy. I tried to stay low so that I didn't disturb anyone. Man, it's always been my peace, kinda like a meditation for me. Nothing else matters when I'm singing. That evening, the doctor reached out to me again. He said, *Hey, Joe, it sounds like you have a fan club. A couple ladies on the floor heard you singing today and were requesting you come back next week. I hope you can cut out a brief gap in your schedule to make a few sick ladies' days. "*

Man, I was thrilled. The next week I showed up with my suit on, guitar and a fresh haircut. I was ready to sing for the people!" Once I got there, there were no people waiting on me. I searched for the doctor to find out where my mystery fans were, but they were non-existent that day. As I was about to leave, a lady that was across the room from where I was last week yelled out to me."

"Excuse me, sir!"

"I slowed down and peaked my head in her room. Yes?"

"Are you here for me? The doctor told me he had a performer that would put on a show for me the same way my daddy used to." The small older lady smiled.

"Now, I wasn't sure how this lady's dad used to play, but I per-formed for her in her room that day for hours. Songs I hadn't sung in years were just coming to me. I continued doing this for weeks. She said it gave her something to look forward to every week, and to be totally honest, she gave me a reason as well. Maybe a month would go by before they finally discharged the little lady. I would seek her information to follow her, but it just never really worked out for me to go to her home and perform."

"Meanwhile, I had completely forgotten about my dire diagnosis. I had a visit scheduled with the doctor that I was looking forward to. I was hoping he had a new patient for me to sing to."

As the doctor entered the room, he asked, "How are you feeling?"

"Well, I'm feeling great, doctor. I'm ready for a new patient to sing to."

The doctor laughed. "I was speaking about your health, but I see you feel the same way your test results read. Which is great. Looks like a bit of purpose has extended your lifespan. The numbers I read a month ago showed you only had so much time to live. I honestly thought it would be weeks."

"Am I healed?" I asked the doctor.

"No, you are healing, and I hope you continue healing for as long as possible. The body is an interesting vehicle. Its magic fuel is purpose, and you, my friend, have found your purpose. No matter the circumstances, you must live your life in your purpose in order to stay alive."

"Now, I'm not sure if he meant to stay alive literally or figuratively, but I took the message to heart. I've been waking up everyday living my purpose and pursuing my aims. I've done so many things that I never had the courage to do since singing for the little lady at the hospital. Along the way, I have learned a few things.

- Do not wait for the perfect place or time to live your purpose.

- Your purpose is not a place.

- Your purpose can be found in your fear or desires. I feared never getting the chance to live out my desire of performing.

- Often your purpose will not be clear, and it will be hidden by a greater issue. My urge to sing before I die sparked the courage to do more.

- Your purpose should not be fixed on one thing. In order to live your purpose, you must accept that life is forever changing but your mindset should not. There's a purpose within every situation. You should pursue your purpose within every environment.

- Release your attachment to results. There's been times since the hospital where I've sung my song and received negative feedback. I've had people boo me and tease me. They have no clue that I'm singing to stay alive, but that's not my worry. I'm doing this for me solely. Selfishly.

"I dress up and go full out in performances. I do this as a reminder that the most important person in the world will be there. That person is always me. The energy that you exude is contagious. Negative energy attracts negative people and positivity attracts positive. Now, not that good things don't negative people, nor does it mean positive people can't experience the bad parts of life. This is a mindset. You can see the same picture with a different perspective. The glass is half full versus half empty. My diagnosis could have shattered me, but it made me more alive. I had been living an unconscious life prior to the day I got my test results. The foods I was eating to satisfy my cravings had now become a deliberate way to nourish myself. My sleeping habits changed, as I realized in order to get the most out of my day, I needed eight hours of sleep. Previously I was lucky to get five or six hours."

"I'm not sure how much longer I got to live, but honestly speaking, I never knew. None of us know, but I know the life I'm living now is way more rewarding than the one previously tied to every title, judgment and fear. I'm alive and living every day."

The old man left Rory with these words:

"Live in your purpose, and you will realize the energy you are generating is magnetic. You will attract the people who are here to serve you and the ones who need to be served. You, my friend, seem to be one who needed to be served this message today."

Who decides if a person can or cannot sing?

I ask the question.

Why not get up and sing?

If the act of singing itself is one that is subjectively measured.

Who decides good or bad?

Does it really matter if the voice sounds the way they want?

Or should we just be happy for the person using their voice?

1 in 3 individuals choose a career, mate and lifestyle based on the assumed outcome or perception.

Most defy the murky direction that unlocks the hearts and follow the more assuring path in hopes of a positive outcome.

Limited but assured by vanity at the least.

This is a common and logical approach to life.

Do what looks best, your life will look like it's perfect. Even if it kills you.

Killing you softly, like smoke seeping from the cracks of a door.

The path of the unknown is dark and fearful.

Running through the smoke, toward the fire.

Burned by judgment but free from the trap of fear.

The labels of perfection and the measuring stick of good or bad end.

Give me my gold star for trying

Although the need for accountability is there.

Is a misspelled word more important than the word itself?

Is it the result or the effort that matters most?

The trap of the heart begins with the mind.

To free it we must go through the door where the smoke seeps through.

The heart is there.

Every human has a unique vocation or duty to share their truth through whatever vessel placed before them. It's not always the vessel we desire, as the story above points out. The old man's vessel was the rare disease. In search of your vocation, you must be able to accept both the good and the bad as a gift. There's a message behind every story, but we must first accept the story as it is. By acknowledging your afflictions, you strip the power it has away. Stand up, face it and sit with it until it works for you.

Chapter 15: Accept

Accept your now but pursue your AIM

The Biggest Fish in the Sea

There's a story about a fish who always heard these stories about the ocean. He spent most of his life dreaming and searching for it. He went on and on obsessing over it. He was tired of where he was. He swam through lakes, ponds and seas. He was fixed on getting to the ocean.

One day a storm ripped through the sea where the fish was traveling. He had no control of his direction. The storm caused major floods. The waters rose so high that one could not separate the lake from the pond. As the storm cleared out and fish floated upstream, he ran across a school of big fish he had never seen. He asked, "Who are you and where are we?"

"We are fish, and we are in water," they replied.

The fish replied, "I know you are fish, and I know we are in water, but I'm asking what type of water is this? Are you guys from the ocean?"

"What is the ocean?" the big fish asked

Frustrated, the fish said, "It's the largest body of water in the world!"

"Oh yes, this is a very large body of water but wouldn't any amount of water that you are in be pretty large to you? Why would you need to seek greater waters if you have waters you are already in?"

Fish replied, "Well, I've always heard that the ocean water is the best and the sea life is amazing. I've swum for months just to have a flood wash everything together."

Big Fish replied, "Months to get to more water? What did you see along the way?"

The fish paused. "Nothing great," he said.

Fish described the days and nights swimming toward the ocean. There were many different kinds of life in the waters. He shared stories of encounters that were chilling; he shared stories of beauty and joy. The big fish listened.

"I did all of that just to get here to reach more water," the fish said.

Big Fish began swimming in the opposite direction.

"Where are you going?" Little fish asked.

"I'm going downstream to the lakes, rivers and ponds. I want to experience the waters the same way you have!"

> **Acceptance should never be confused with complacent. Every day you must have an aim to pursue in order to insure happiness.**

We have all come to grips that the sun rises and falls. The seasons change from winter to spring, summer to fall. We may not like it, but we understand there is life and death as well.

We realize life is a mere series of opposites cycling continuously, yet immeasurable levels of energy are spent trying to avoid one of the most necessary opposites in our lives. This opposite is the feeling of DISCOMFORT. Yes, a very broad and not-so-sexy way of putting it, but when we look at it deeper, we see that behind every fear, doubt, judgment or hesitation lies this feeling of discomfort.

We have all been here in our lives. Palms sweating, sometimes a little shaky and even hard to breathe. There are many reactions to being in uncomfortable situations. Boy can it be nerve wrecking, and it's anything but the luxurious headspace that we'd rather be in. The easiest thing to do is to run from it. Hide and never face the agony again. Unfortunately, you cannot run from that which is within you. At some point discomfort will present itself regardless if you like it. Pain is a given, suffering is an option. Notice I shared the symptoms instead of searching for a label. Remember, it is the label that kills the soul most often not the issue itself.

What we want to do instead is learn to accept the current moment as the only moment. You treat your life with the same flexibility that you find with the weather. When it is winter, you wear a coat. You grab an umbrella when it rains; you take off layers in the spring, and you grab your shorts in the summer.

It makes little sense to sit in the joy of 80 degree weather and pray that it stays that way. You've found acceptance in the sun rising and setting. You are at peace with flow. Let's accept the Sun and Moon within yourself.

The fish had all the right to pursue the ocean because the ocean represents more life that he hasn't seen. What the fish failed to realize is that what he desired the most was already before his eyes.

Gratitude is being appreciative for the life that lies before you.

Embrace Discomfort

The great misconception is that we should do things that make us comfortable in a world where we have no control over most things besides our reactions. We can waste more than half of our life waiting for ideal circumstances.

I've heard it for years: *I can't meditate because my mind won't turn off.*

We want the mind turned on, actually. We want to see everything that is, so that we can realize everything that isn't. The thoughts that swirl in our heads can be like a tornado. A head full of distractions makes it seem completely impossible to sit still. It's annoying, or shall I say it's uncomfortable, to sit through. The instinct is to get up, to get away from the tornado of thoughts. However, as we all know, you can't outrun a tornado; you must wait until it has passed or find your way to the eye of the storm. The calmest place is the center. With practice, you develop the ability to find calm amid any storm life delivers. This is critical for your sanity in the real world.

You are now equipped to observe the fluctuations of your day the same way you observed the fluctuations in your mediation. Sit with what is instead of where you want to be. Acceptance of your now will allow you to embrace life's challenges as forever changing parts of life. It's said that the practice begins when things get difficult. I like to believe Rory's life began on the tough day he watched his mom take her last gasp of breath.

We have no control over the circumstances of the world but we control how we perceive it. We have the option to view the glass as half full or half empty. We hold the key to freedom within, but we must first acknowledge the trap.

Moving toward the things that make you uncomfortable frees you.

Yoga Is the Lens Through Which You See Within

It is extremely common for the person beginning their yoga journey to speak about what they lack. They use negative words to describe themselves, such as "I'm always tight, I can't focus, I have no balance, I am old, fat," etc.

We want to use the practice to see what is instead of what isn't. The stability of a balancing pose is within the mind, not the body. One who has mastered balancing on one foot is no more stable than the person falling to the ground, if the mind is rabid.

In the same breath, the person falling side to side but remaining calm as they try to gain stability has in fact found the mental balance that we seek.

You are not broken; you do not need to be fixed. The body responds to the words and thoughts you create within it. Start by changing the words you use when speaking about your body. This is not a simple task, as they conditioned us from early childhood to focus on labeling things as good or bad instead of simply allowing things to be. Not that you should not identify feelings and thoughts. I actually encourage you to do this. My suggestion is that you stray away from identifying yourself as these thoughts or feelings.

We achieve this through deliberate practice. From the outside looking in, a person would look at yoga as an opportunity to gain flexibility, and you will. They may also see it as a space to gain strength, and this is also likely. One may even look at yoga as an opportunity to gain ultimate liberation from stress. These are all accurate assumptions. However, the first and most important thing you gain from yoga is your ability to observe, identify and accept your current truth while practicing postures.

Yes, each forward fold tells a different story, each backbend unfolds another truth. It's not the shape that we seek, it's the stars we see along the way. So begin by telling yourself, *I'm not tight, I have found my resistance* and *I'm not weak, I've found my edge*. There is no age, weight, gender or ailment that can defy this universal truth. If you can find your personal edge without attachment to the result, then you can attain liberation.

Chapter 16: Living vs Surviving

THE OLD MAN learned to acknowledge and smell his flowers after receiving the worst news of his life. He realized that the days he had remaining were numbered, so waiting for sweeter results might have left him parting earth without ever living out his desires. If we are honest, we would acknowledge that none of us really know our expiration date. We should all appreciate the now.

Rory began thinking more and more about his own path. *Am I really living in my purpose? Do I have to get a death sentence in order to really discover the fruit of my life? Aren't we all given a death sentence upon birth?*

At age 19, Rory sat at the doctor's office with his dad every week for eight hours at a time. His dad was facing his second bout with prostate cancer. Just five years earlier, Rory had watched his dad struggle with the aftermath of having his prostate removed. The monster had returned to his bones this time. Chemotherapy was the remedy to maintain but not cure him. The doctor would determine each week how much therapy he needed. Some weeks they were there eight hours, and other weeks it could be as much as ten hours of slow drip therapy in the cold hospital. I'll let Rory explain the days in chemo.

My dad rarely spoke about having cancer. It was almost as if it didn't exist. He changed nothing. He was a master masker of his feelings. And he was not about to let the C word expose him as weak. He suddenly wore smiles he had never displayed in his years prior to the disease. We've had a relationship my entire life, but this was different. He shared more, and we laughed more than we ever did. It was like cancer was bringing us closer together.

Rory enjoyed the days at chemo ironically. The hospital was like stepping into an episode of Cheers. Everyone knew your name there. There were over 50 people in the same clinic every week with the same diagnosis. They came in all races and ages. Some came in wheelchairs and others on walkers. Rory's dad still had the strength to walk in but often had to be wheeled out as the therapy stripped away any juice he had left.

Despite the circumstances, the courageous patients made light of the moment every week. They'd throw on a smile and confess life is great if you ask them *how they are feeling*. Cancer had slowly turned Rory's dad to a frail shell of himself but his personality remained the same. He was the jokester. He made sure the entire clinic knew when he was coming in.

The nurses knew his jokes were his way of covering up his fears. No matter how inappropriate, they'd still give him a giggle, wondering how far he'd take it each day.

"What dirty joke you got for us today, Mr. Powers?" the nurse asked as she inserted the IV into his fate veins.

With a grin, he gave the people of the clinic what they asked for. "What do you call a blind gynecologist?"

"Hmmmm. A blind gynecologist. I don't know, Mr. Powers."

"That's a lip reader." He said with a devilish grin.

Laughter filled the room, creating an environment if only for one moment where the cold clinical room didn't feel so bad. Rory laughed as well but he could see through the facade his dad was presenting.

I watched him use his sense of humor to mask the fear of his life fading away. My dad avoided talking in depth about the ending of life. The disease that entered his body had become a bridge for our relationship.

He would tell me stories that I had never heard about him, my mom, and even me as a kid. The once concealed soul was giving me what I had desired for years. Chemotherapy had become the ultimate connector. Eight full hours of conversation.

One day in the middle of the summer, the doctor walked into the cold, air-conditioned office to do her monthly update on how the cancer was responding to the treatments.

"Mr. Powers, are you still smoking cigarettes?"

"Hell yeah, I'm still smoking. What's gonna happen? Cancer? I already got that."

She had no rebuttal. "Mr. Powers, you have to stop smoking to give yourself a chance to fight this."

"Okay, Doc, I hear you. I'm going to quit after today."

He never quit.

The drain that the chemo put on his body was tough to witness, but not nearly as tough as the moment the doctor entered the room with a stone face.

Fresh into telling a joke, Rory's dad looked up.

"What's up, doc?"

"Mr. Powers, I'm ending your chemotherapy treatments."

"Oh okay! So the cancer is gone?! We beat it?"

"No, Mr. Powers, unfortunately, the cancer has spread more. I'm ending the chemotherapy because the cancer has spread so much that it is better to have comfort in your last days than to keep the treatments going."

Lost in her words and waiting for clarity, Rory asked, "*So, what are you saying?*"

"Unfortunately, it's looking like your dad only has a short time left to live. You'll see drastic changes in his body. I will refer a hospice nurse that will help make the process comfortable for you."

Rory and his dad both sat in disbelief.

I'll never forget the long pause, followed by my dad saying:

"Damn… that's it man. I guess that's it."

The frog in my throat had me holding back tears and trying to think of the best thing to say as I could for the first time, see the fear in my daddy's eyes.

The downward spiral happened just as the doctor explained. She gave a bleak process that could take months, weeks, or just days. In Rory's dad's case, it was just 11 days. Every day went just as the doctor predicted. He suddenly lost the ability to swallow food. He would chew the same bite for minutes but could not swallow it down. His body ached unbearably; the doctor came to visit and discovered his pelvis had shattered from lying in the bed.

Unfucking believable to think a person doing absolutely nothing could have so many things going wrong so fast.

They gave him liquid morphine to manage the pain he was having because there was nothing they could do for his pelvis; he was too frail at that point.

That liquid morphine may have eased the pain, but it also took away his brain. He was never the same after that.

The home nurse was there to deliver the drugs.

"He will be more comfortable in about 30 minutes," she said.

I was beginning to think comfortable was the buzzword for "dead to the world."

Almost immediately, the wheels flew off. He slept for 20 hours straight.

I went in several times a day to see if his belly was still rising and falling as he laid on his back. When he woke up, there was nothing said. Unresponsive, he just gazed at the ceiling. Still, I would pretend nothing was wrong.

"Alright dad, I'm heading to work. Mama will be here in a minute."

Even though Rory's parents had divorced 15 years prior, Rory's mama still had his back—or maybe it was Rory she was there for. Regardless, she was there to give Rory a break in caring for his dad.

The days would go so long, but the changes were happening so fast. After two days motionless, his dad started talking again. Rory jumped up in excitement, but Rory's dad wasn't saying anything directly. Still looking at the ceiling, he was talking, but it was almost like sleep talking. He was reciting experiences from his life.

"Nah, man, you gotta go to 43rd Street and get cigarettes… then go to the bank and get money out for me…"

He was mumbling words from his 65 years of life. A couple times he would say things that were familiar to Rory. This went on non-stop for two days straight. Rory had given up on telling the doctor anything.

Only god knows what type of comforting drug she had under her sleeve next. I told her we didn't need anymore morphine either.

The third day, as Rory prepared to leave for work, he did his typical pretend-like-everything-is-normal "see ya later." This time, to Rory's surprise, his dad looked at him with a big smile.

"Rory! What are you doing here, man?"

"Oh, I'm here to be with you, daddy. Just to keep you company."

His dad closed his eyes with a smile still on his face.

"Okay."

Rory had been holding it together, but this broke the dam open. He burst into tears. Uncontrollably he stuffed his head into his pillow sobbing. After 65 years of hard, his dad finally softened those last days. They were so much alike. Neither was interested in expressing their true love they had for one another. The smile and the peace Rory witnessed in that simple "okay" was enough love to fill his heart for a lifetime. He could not stop crying. This was years of wearing a mask that was finally removed. Who would have thought "okay" could be so powerful?

If okay was the last word, I was okay with that as well.

Exactly one day later, Rory woke up to his dad completely stiff. No life left in him.Death was inevitable but the paralyzing effect of the liquid morphine that was given to make him comfortable also took away his joy, care and urge to keep moving. It taught Rory the greatest lessons his dad had ever taught him.

1. **Movement is 100% essential in life. No matter what you are going through, you must get up and move daily.**

2. **Pain is a necessary part of life. Suffering is optional. The overload in drugs made the sensations associated with Rory's father's pain nonexistent. It also stripped him of a reason to move.**

3. **Life is unpredictable so say it now, do it now, feel it now. Rory's dad dropped a barrier in his last days that opened Rory's heart for the future. The smile after he realized Rory was there with him will in Rory's heart forever.**

I stayed with him those final 11 days. The stories he told me those last days trumped any advice he had given me over the years. He was more vulnerable than I had ever heard, telling me about things I had never heard. He was speaking his truth, and I was there to be an ear.

"Hell yeah I'm scared, man. I don't want to die."

The ironic thing was that they diagnosed him with incurable cancer. Treatment to manage was the only option. But it wasn't until they gave him an actual time frame that the slide began. Doctors are humans, as we all know, and they are merely reading results of tests and giving their best recommendations based on what they see. But you can't help but wonder how different things would have been if Rory's dad had a doctor like the old singing man.

The doctors had different perspectives on life—one which suggests you should spend your last days doing all the things that you were uncomfortable doing. Experiencing the things that you feared most. While Rory's dad's doctor prescribed medications so that he would be comfortable on the way to heaven's gates, the comfortable path led to a brisk death which still brought intense discomfort. The path the singing man took was uncomfortable to begin but led to a sense of liberation and more life. The old man found his purpose within the belly of the greatest fear of death itself.

Chapter 17: Rory Story

Rory Sits with It

After talking with the old singing man, Rory began heading back to his room. He had a ton on his mind to unpack, and the walk back to the hotel was much slower.

The questions in his head caused a tornado of thoughts.

Why aren't all doctors speaking life into their patients instead of death? My dad had the exact opposite experience with his doctor. She basically sent the undertaker over to help him die easier.

Being a witness of death and a listener of life, Rory realized at that moment that we all have a choice to live or to die.

My dad was dying before death, while the singing man was living before he died.

By the time Rory made it back to the hotel, he checked his phone and saw he had a text from the lady he'd helped with her bags earlier.

"Hey what are you doing? I'm thinking about grabbing food and taking my baby to the beach. You can join us if you're still roaming around lonely." She said,

Who said I was lonely? I'm actually enjoying myself. Besides, it's kinda odd linking up with a lady with a little baby with her. Time for an excuse.

"*Hey, I'm about to take a yoga class. I'll hit you up afterward.*"

Just like the loner that he was, Rory blew off his best chance of having company on this trip.

Rory started heading toward the yoga studio. He saw on the schedule that there was an ashtanga fundamentals class happening soon. He had about 15 minutes to get there, so he made his way down the oceanfront with a nice jog. The studio was up the street from the restaurant he'd eaten at earlier, but Rory was having a tough time locating it. The yogis led him to the space before, but this time there were none in sight.

Rory walked around for a minute before he finally gave the studio a call. The lady who'd greeted him earlier answered the phone.

"Hello, yes, there is a fundamentals class going on now, but it's only a 30-minute class, and you're already 15 minutes late."

Figures.

"Oh wow, okay, when is your next class? I met you earlier."

"Oh, is this Rory?!"

"Yes, it is!"

"I was hoping you would make it. If you come tomorrow, I will take good care of you. Promise me you will come tomorrow, Rory!"

"Okay, yes, I will come tomorrow. What time?"

"Come at 10 a.m. sharp. I will send you directions so that you don't get lost."

Rory was excited to have something to do tomorrow but now had nowhere to go today. He looked at his phone then replied to the message from the lady he'd met at the hotel.

"Hey, are you guys still going to the beach?"

It's Never Too Late to Begin

Rory started walking back toward the hotel still thinking about the conversation he'd had with the old singing man.

Is there anything that I want to do that I haven't? I've never wanted to sing or do anything crazy, honestly. Never cared to be rich and famous. I don't know what I would want to do before I die.

Rory was stuck trying to think of something to do before he died. What he was missing was the liberation the old man had gained just by pursuing something. It does not have to be your loftiest dream for you to pursue it. It can be the simplest things that make the greatest impact.

Rory eventually made it back to the hotel when his phone rang from a Flint, Michigan area code. A loud woman's voice came through the other end.

"Where you at, man? I've been trying to invite you to come chill at the pool with me instead of the beach. You must have found a new friend already."

"*OH HEY! Nah, my phone was on silent, my bad.*"

"Well, if you ain't doing shit, come to my pool. And bring some water, it's hot down here!"

Wow, this lady is so damn demanding. You would have assumed I've known her for decades.

But Rory wasn't doing anything else. He grabbed a couple waters, tossed them in his book bag and headed out. The hotel she stayed at was only 5 mins away from Rory's. In no time he made it to the hotel's pool.

"Finally! I thought you went on a nature walk again. We were about to pass out waiting for these waters." The Flint Girl blurted as Rory arrived.

Seeing the cute smirk on her face made her loud and aggressive approach more digestible. Rory smiled.

"You're hella bossy, ma'am. You couldn't ask someone who works here for a bottle of water?"

With a smile, she looked away.

"I knew you'd look better bringing it."

Whew, that was a direct shot there. Not sure if I should hit on her back or if the baby she's holding would find that disrespectful flirting with his moms.

Rory smiled back as he pulled up a chair.

"So what have y'all been doing?"

"Nothing, just chilling here. There's not much I can do with a six-month-old baby with me, but he's my road dog and I just wanted some warm weather. How about you?"

"Oh, same here. I've really just been hanging around since I saw you earlier. I ran across this old guy singing, and I ended up having a really good conversation with him."

She looked at Rory, perplexed

"An old guy singing? A homeless man?"

"Nah, he wasn't homeless, he actually had a career and family. He said he was out there singing because that was his long-burning desire."

"Oh, you like weird stuff, huh?"

"It wasn't weird. Have you ever seen street performers?"

"Yeah, man I'm just joking with you. I love street shows, too," she said. "But we are about to get in the water, you coming?"

"Nah, I don't feel like getting in the water. I'll watch y'all and grab a drink."

"Why not? You can't swim?"

"Nope, actually I can't."

"Why not? Your big, grown ass is not afraid of water, are you?"

"I have no reason to be afraid of water. I live on land. Throw me in the ocean, then yes, of course I would be afraid. But I never learned as a kid, so as I got older I left it alone."

"You're never too old to learn anything. Once you stop learning, you stop growing. At that point you may as well die."

"Well, damn, that's pretty drastic, but I get what you mean. That's actually what me and the old singing man were discussing. He asked me to think of my deepest desires and to live them out. I couldn't think of anything. But learning to swim would be cool."

"Yes! They actually have swim lessons here tomorrow. I'm putting my baby in it. You should see if they have adult lessons."

"Really? I'm only here for one more day, there's no way they can teach me to swim in that short of time."

"It doesn't matter if you learn or not. You just said this was one of your desires, so why wait? Do that shit now. I'll call for you."

Hot damn, who sent this bossy-ass lady to take over my trip?

As she picked up her phone and walked away, her baby looked at Rory from his stroller with a smile.

"Damn, little fella, you have a hell of a mama on your hands. Good luck with that."

As Rory was laughing, The Flint Girl finally got a hold of someone on the phone.

"Hello, hi, I have swimming lessons for my son tomorrow. My boyfriend wants to take an adult lesson. Oooooh okay, yeah, that's fine, he will be okay. He never learned to swim as a kid. We will see you tomorrow." She laughed through the phone, then hung up. She walked back over with a big grin on her face. "Looks like you will be learning to swim tomorrow."

Laughing and nervous, Rory said, *"Oh my god, you are so crazy."*

"What? I'm helping you out! You said you want to live out your desires, so there you have it. Time to face your fears."

Through empathy, we discover how listening can liberate us from the chains of our autobiographical experiences, freeing us to enter the realm of what is, as opposed to being consumed by what isn't. This opens the door to authentic relationships and growth.

Your story may be unique, but the feelings associated are not. This is not intended to devalue anyone's story. Instead it empowers you by being able to accept and understand others as they are. There's nothing more satisfying than a person accepting you for your flaws and all. One of the greatest empathizers can be seen in the Kanye West Donda documentary. The love his mom showed was one of patience, grace and acceptance. As Kanye vented about not being taken seriously as a rapper, she said to him, "Okay, Kanye, I know what you mean, your passion will always shine through. That won't change. But you can't force people to see, feel and hear the way you do. You must continue to be you and allow them the same grace to see that you have so much more to offer the world."

Most people don't want your pity, and no one really needs it. What they do need is to feel like you understand them not just intellectually but emotionally and energetically. The assurance that Kanye's mother gave him just by saying she heard him is what empowers us.

Empathy is not agreeing or disagreeing. Empathy is hearing from a perspective that is not your own without casting judgment or opinion. This allows the speaker to be. This allows the listener to see.

Sometimes We Just Need an Ear to Talk To. No Judgment or Advice.

God has a way of placing the right people in our lives at the right time. Rory and Flint Girl's conversations carried all the way through the night. He learned about her fears of being a baby mama again 17 years after having her first child.

She confessed, "I was afraid of love for so long because I didn't want the label of *baby mama* again. I want to be a wife but…"

She stopped as her eyes began to water.

"What are some things you fear? Besides swimming of course." She burst into laughter.

"*Hmmm. I don't know what I fear.*" Rory replied.

I feared not measuring up. Anything that required effort I feared because I didn't want to be judged if I failed. This fear kept me from committing fully in relationships for fear of having my heart broken. This kept me from starting my own business in fear of it not working and having to face people who believed in me. This kept me driving a car that I didn't want because I feared it being repossessed or stolen. My fears run deep but I wasn't ready to share them.

They went back and forth, baring their souls and creating connections based solely on listening. The interesting thing is that they were exposing great desire within each fear. They hadn't realized it, but the trust that they were developing as they revealed their stories was creating self-acceptance that would be foundational for the mindset both needed to pursue their aims. The softening was happening for both.

No physical activity could happen with the baby there. Rory decided not to get a drink since Flint Girl was unable to enjoy one with him, due to breastfeeding.

For the first time I was experiencing a connection that was not tied solely to the end goal. Although I had banging her on my mind, I didn't see it as a possibility with the baby here. Hell, I still had no clue where the baby's dad was or anything.

Instead of getting lost in where this could go, they decided to enjoy it for what it was. They sat by the pool until the sun set, talking and sharing stories.

"Wow, look, the sun is setting. Let's walk over to the beach! We've been sitting here for hours," Flint Girl said.

Rory easily agreed, as he wasn't looking forward to going back to his lonely room.

Listen to Me

The baby had finally fallen asleep at this point. He didn't put up much fuss as it was, but now he lay in his stroller completely asleep as they made their way over through the high winds gusting from the ocean. It wasn't the warmest of nights, but it beat January in Detroit.

"*Whew! It's a lot cooler over here than the pool was,*" Rory blurted out.

"Man, you will be okay. I have an extra blanket."

She rolled the stroller up the sand hill. Rory had come accustomed to her bossy ways by now. She found a spot right in the center of the fire-orange sun. The sky was reflecting a yellow, orange and purple glaze, but it took mere moments for it to turn completely black and showered by stars. They continued talking.

"So tell me about your love life," she implored.

"*My love life? There isn't one. I was with a girl for a couple years, and that didn't work out. Ever since then it's been a crapshow of women coming in and out of my life. Every time I meet someone I like, they do something that turns me off.*"

"Turn you off how? Are you one of those stuck-up guys who needs his woman doing all this unrealistic shit?" she laughed.

"*Nah, I'm easy, actually. As long as you don't do anything odd or blatantly disrespectful, I'm good.*"

"So what do you consider disrespect? Is that why you and your girl broke up?"

"*Yeah, basically. She was mean as hell. I couldn't joke with her or do anything without it making her upset. She would go off over the simplest shit.*"

"So you left her because she was mean? She couldn't have been too mean, you had to have liked something about her."

"Nah, it kept getting worse, so I kindly encouraged her to leave."

"Leave? Y'all lived together?! Man, you definitely loved something about her to have her living in your house."

"I did like her a lot at first. She was cool to talk to after my dad passed away. We had good conversations and fun when we were just dating. As soon as I became her boyfriend, things changed. Almost like the title boyfriend gave her a new sense of entitlement over me. It got worse after she moved in. "

"Oh yeah, I know that scenario all too well. It's cool and fun at the beginning, but as soon as the titles come, so does the leash and the asshole attitude."

"Exactly! It's like people want an object instead of a companion. I'd hate for someone to change me."

"So how'd you get her to leave?"

"I got up one day and told her I was going out of town. She didn't like me doing anything without her, I knew it would have her boiling. I stayed gone for a week."

"So she left while you were gone?"

"Yep, I got back home and the house was stripped. No curtains, sheets or dishes. The only thing she left me was a pile of shit in the toilet."

"Shit?! Wait, what do you mean?!" The Flint Girl laughed.

"She literally took everything out of the house and took a shit in the toilet and didn't flush it. Shit was stuck on the inside of the toilet, and I couldn't clean it because she took the toilet brush with her, too."

"Well, damn!" She was laughing hysterically now. "That's what I'm talking about, sis. Shit on his ass since he wants to go. I need to take some notes from her."

"Okay, okay, calm down, you don't even know her. You're supposed to be on my side."

"Nah, y'all men be out of control, so we gotta stick together and shit on y'all sometimes."

"I guess so. What's your story? What man has you shitting on us?"

"My story is just like most. I met a guy. He's great, and just as soon as I got comfortable, he switched up. I've had two long-term relationships. Three kids. The first was when I was in high school, a mistake but a blessing even still. My daughter, I had with my then-husband when I was 23 years old. Then, after 16 years of having a cold heart, I finally softened for a man who promised me the world. Until, *boom*, my soon-to-be 40 year old ass gets pregnant. Now shit has changed, of course."

"Changed like how?"

"He just changed. The way he talked to me and the things that he would do. I don't know, it's just different. Everything derives around work now. Like he thinks I'm supposed to just sit in the house all day and do nothing."

"Sounds like y'all are still together. Did you tell him how you feel?"

"Yes, I tell his ass every day that I'm not no damn mother goose sitting in the house waiting on him everyday. That's why I got the fuck up and came out of town without him."

"Sounds like we have a little in common here. You're doing the exact same thing that I did to get my ex to leave me. The thing I wonder is, if you really want him to leave, or if you just want him to hear you. I've only known you for a few hours, but I can almost bet that your delivery probably caused him to push back instead of listening."

"Nah, my delivery is good. It's his dumb ass, always talking about how else is his son gonna eat if he doesn't work."

"Yeah, that's what I mean. He's thinking about the baby but forgetting about you. Sometimes we need a levelheaded conversation. One

where both parties can be heard without a rebuttal. Then swapping and letting the opposite person speak."

"You Dr. Phil now?"

"Nope, we did this exercise in a class I took on empathic listening. The idea is to listen with your eyes and heart but without agreeing or disagreeing with any statements. Simply allow yourself to see the opposing perspective."

"That kinda makes sense, I guess, but it's hard. I've been through a lot in my life. Men try to control with their money or by getting you pregnant. I've had this happen to me one too many times. Now I can almost smell it coming. All y'all are the same, I swear."

"What do you mean you've been through this your entire life?"

"The control. It started when I was only 16 years old. My boyfriend at the time was 19. He had a car and already graduated high school. He was cute and had way more money than any of the boys in high school. He would pick me up from school. I felt so grown, walking to my boyfriend's car while everyone else was walking to their mama car. I loved that shit. As the school year went on, it became a not-so-cool obligation. I'd have days where I'd want to hang out with my friends after school, go to football and basketball games. He would get so upset saying shit like, *Why do you want to hang out with them little ass kids? I'm trying to treat you like a queen but you want to ride a bus with babies."*

"It was so annoying. I didn't want to make him mad, so I skipped all my high school activities. It was always a problem, one way or another, every time something came up that he couldn't be involved in. The icing on the cake came my 12th grade year. My school had a strict rule about no outside guests for our senior prom. I told him about this months before to prepare him. He mostly ignored my hints that I planned to go. It wasn't until my mom took me dress shopping when it set in that I would be going even though he wasn't permitted to attend."

"He said, *"So you're really going to this prom without your man? Who do you think you are going with then?* I remember telling him I was going alone, probably, or maybe my best friend Clay, just for the pictures. He knew Clay and also knew nothing would ever happen between me and him, yet it still drove him ballistic. We argued in his car for so long that the windows fogged up. He made his typical threats to leave me for someone more mature. Someone with grown shit to do."

"I said, *Go fuck with you an old bitch! I'll be sure to find a young dick to jump on prom night.* Just as fast as my words came out, his hand came up as he slapped me. It was the first time he'd put his hands on me but definitely not the last. I tried my best to fight him back. I scratched, kicked and clawed at him. He eventually overpowered me, and with his hand around my throat, he said, *bitch if you ever say anything about another nigga's dick, I'll kill you.*"

"I don't know if it was the young age or what, but that made me so Goddamned horny. Before I knew it, my panties were down, while he still had his hand around my throat. The tighter he grabbed my neck, the more I wanted him. He never let go of my neck as he started fucking me. He was calling me all types of names, and I liked it. It was that day he got me pregnant. He never pulled out. He looked me right in my eye as he came. It was so stupid of me. I let him do it. I was in the moment. To this day, I believe he did it on purpose in hopes of ruining my prom plans."

"Wow. So did you go to prom?"

"No. I was five months pregnant by the time of prom. I was too embarrassed to show my face at the school once I started showing. My mom convinced the principal to allow me to finish my final semester from home. I didn't even walk across the stage for graduation. I missed all the stuff that a kid remembers forever simply because I didn't want to make a weak man upset. I vowed then to never ever let that shit happen again. If I want to do something, I'm gonna do it and no man is gonna control me."

"Damn, that makes total sense now. Something like that would make it hard to trust again. How long did you and your kids' dad last together?"

"Too long. He would not let me breathe after I had that baby. It was like hell on earth. I loved my baby but I could not do anything without him checking to see where I was at. He wanted my baby to be a weight that kept me chained to the house so nobody on earth could see me but him."

"Yikes. I'm guessing you were thrilled when you finally got away."

"Yeah, after I shot his ass!"

"You shot him?!"

"Man, hell yeah. He kept putting his hands on me."

"Did he die?"

"Noooo! What, are you scared of me now? I'm not a killer, Ro," she said, laughing. "I just can't understand why men think they can control you. I don't need a man for money, food or a house. I got all of that myself, so I'm fine all by myself with my kids."

"Yeah, I hear what you are saying, and I totally understand it, but from the sound of it, it seems like you already had your mind set once you began dating him. Of course I'm certain there is more to it than you are saying, but for the most part you've said that you knew he would become controlling. While from a man's perspective it sounds like he is trying to protect, provide and care for you. Now, he may not be aware that you have experienced the trauma from high school."

"Trauma? Man, that wasn't no trauma. The boy slapped me, we fucked, and I got pregnant. I wouldn't call it trauma. Just a fucked up part of my life that I'd rather leave in the past. But yeah, I told him about it when I told him about my oldest kid."

"Okay, he knows about how you got pregnant, but does he know how this has tarnished your view on love and relationships? Meaning you can't be properly loved if the person you are with has no idea of the things that you are protecting yourself from. Think about it this way: If you cross your arms over your chest to protect your heart, I will not be able to hurt you. In the same sense, if you keep your arms crossed over your chest, I will never be able to hug and love you, either."

Rory and Flint Girl shared similar fears in regards to love and relationships. Neither has reached a point where they are able to recognize this seed in their soil. The only way to love freely is to embrace the possibility of both outcomes happening. You will not die from heartbreak. Yet stripping yourself of the opportunity to love and to be loved can leave you living in a life of misery. The protection that we build over years of being hurt creates a wall that prevents the vibration from coming through. In order to experience true love, we must be vulnerable enough to lower the shield and bare the soul. Keep in mind the most important display of love is the one you show to yourself. It is not tied to a person or thing. Love is an energetic vibration. The more love you give off to the universe, the more love you will attract. This is a practice and will never be perfect. If you practice the perspective of life happening for you, you attract the people who align with your mindset. Once again, it begins with you. Bare your soul to receive the love you deserve. Cover your soul and receive the love people believe you deserve.

"So you want me to go tell my boyfriend that I can't stand him because of the guy that got me pregnant in high school?" Flint Girl says with her nose up.

"*Well not like that*," Rory said, laughing. *I'd say it would be a cool conversation like we are having now, where you tell him just like you just told me that you don't want any man controlling you. Tell him that you missed out on parts of your life due to control. So you have a hard time experiencing any signs of the same tendency. I'm willing to bet that he wasn't aware that he was harming more than helping.*"

"Okay, Dr. Phil. I'm gonna try it, but what about your ass? You're around here with nobody but your damn self. Where's your love at?"

"*Yeah, I have my own shit I'm still digging through. My seed is tied to my mom. I still can't bring myself to let any woman into my life completely. I fear needing them and it being thrown back in my face. My mom was the one person I could rely on for anything.*"

"Oh, see, that's some deep shit for sure. We will have to continue this conversation tomorrow. It's time for the baby and I to get some rest. Go get some rest so that your ass is up early tomorrow for this swim class," she said, laughing.

Swim Day

The next day, Rory woke up to three text messages that were sent late at night.

"Set your alarm for 7 a.m."

"Are you asleep?"

"I can't sleep. You should have just come with us to keep me company."

Just as he was reading, the phone rang.

"Are you up?!" Flint Girl screams through the phone.

"*Yes, ma'am. I'm up.*"

"Good. I didn't get any sleep. The baby woke up at 4 a.m. just when I was falling asleep. So I hope this class wears him out so I can get a nap in."

"Oh, wow. Yes, I just saw your messages. I went right to sleep when I got to the room. I'll meet you at your pool in 20 minutes."

Rory grabbed his book bag and headed out.

Chapter 18: Practice Over Perfection

Becoming

Happiness is a state of mind that can be experienced at any moment. The joy is in *doing* more than in *receiving*. You witness this with a clear vision of your why. Without asking what you are getting, instead ask yourself "what am I becoming?" Your interactions at work, with family, friends, and strangers are opportunities to watch your becoming unfold. Your way out of the trap is uniquely tied to your ability to allow EVERYTHING to contribute to your becoming.

When I began coaching football, we had approximately 40 to 50 kids on the team. This was the case each year for about five years straight. One year, the organization saw a ton of turmoil and lost a lot of kids and coaches, leaving the team with a skimpy 16 kids total. I had the opportunity to leave as the ship was sinking just like the other coaches, but I saw two things in this situation. One, I knew these loyal kids deserved a coach that believed in them. The impact I could make on them if I stayed would be life-changing. Two, this was also an opportunity to watch my becoming unfold. I had a challenge in front of me to get 16 boys to compete for a championship against teams with 40 players on their squad. We had this goal set but we weren't tied to the result.

We weren't chasing a trophy. I took a different approach. My mantra was, "Practice over Perfection." No matter your talent level, size or strength, the one thing I want you to focus on is treating everything like practice. I gave them permission to mess up and make mistakes as much as they needed. We set daily aims that sometimes seemed ridiculous, as the drills had zero to do with football. Yet I knew exactly what my personal aim for them was. I was looking to shape their mentality. Having just 16 boys I could not run the risk of losing a kid because their confidence was shot. My aim was to ensure they could handle success and failure the same way.

The kids trusted my words. I spent weeks focusing on them doing their best at the simple details. Getting in line for warmups took a month to figure out.

"You have 25 seconds to make four lines four yards apart," I yelled. It turned into a frenzy. Nine-year-olds were running in circles as they raced to get lined up in 30 seconds. Every time they didn't complete the task, they had to run a 300 meter lap in less than one minute. Every time they missed, it became more difficult. They were frustrated and often in tears. For two weeks, I sat on the sideline and watched them try to figure it out on their own. I watched as they gained the conditioning both mental and physically. They fought and argued with each other pointing the blame. I allowed them to experience all of the emotions. I continued delivering the same message every day before practice: "Practice over Perfection!"

They finally came to me and said they didn't think it was possible to get aligned in 25 seconds. I smiled and said, "Do your personal best, and everything else will fall into place." As I got off the bench on the sidelines, I told the first boy I saw to come to me. I told him to stand still. I then asked for the second boy to come and asked him to count four yards and stop. I asked the third boy to do the same, and the fourth.

"Now give me three more that can go four yards apart the other direction. Then everyone else falls in line."

I yelled as loud as I could, "Do your personal best, and everything else will fall in place!" They were so caught up in the big picture (the 25 second time)that they missed the most important step of just counting off four yards and standing still.

This is common for most people. We obsess over the task so much that we miss the most critical steps. This drill taught the boys to work together by working on themselves first. They became a well oiled machine as every day after running their lap, they lined themselves up one by one in less than 25 seconds. Defying the thought that it was impossible. As we began inserting football plays they kept the same mindset. They were able to line up and run the plays without fighting each other. When there was a hiccup in a play no one panicked,they had already accepted the practice over perfection mindset. The boys learned the way you do one thing, is the way you do everything.

We were a shock to everyone in the league that season. We won every single game without giving up a single point. Every player on the field realized if they did their best individually, then good would come. They put in the work and attracted the victories. In the first round of the playoffs, we were beat by a much better team, ending our season. The seed had been firmly planted in the boys' soil, though.

Two years later, one of the boys from the team invited me to his honors ceremony at his school. He got on the stage to speak and shared this remarkable story.

"When I was 9, no one wanted to coach our team because there weren't a lot of us. Coach Randall stayed though, he made us do yoga. YOGA?! This is football, and he's teaching us to breathe through difficult moments. He kept making us run laps while saying, "Practice over Perfection! Do your best and the rest will fall into place."

I couldn't stand it, but now I understand.

That season we did really well, but the real benefit came from Coach teaching us to breathe when different emotions came up. I used to get so nervous before tests and forget everything. This year, before every test I did what Coach would tell us before a game. Take a deep breath and treat it like practice. So I did each individual question instead of looking at the entire test."

"Now, this year, I'm on the honor roll for the first time ever! I invited Coach Randall because he has made a positive impact in my life."

That ceremony brought me to tears and gave me confirmation that the seeds were not only planted but also flourishing. The goal for any team is typically a championship. We didn't get the football championship, but I like to believe we had a bunch of stars that we were able to witness in pursuit of the championship. They are continuing to shine to this day.

Each one of the 16 boys from that team is currently in college, and five of them are playing football. I made the impact, just not the one I was expecting. They made an impact on me that I wasn't expecting. The small things you do now can bear lasting fruit in the future.

Your actions contribute directly to what you attract. Your personal development depends on you shifting your mindset to one of action. My karma was taking action for the boys. The boys' karma was taking action for one another. The detachment from the results allowed both of our perspectives to be shifted to one of experience instead of chasing. This is the major key. Enjoy the scenic route as you become your why.

This is a mindset that we will use in our yoga practice as well but before we go there lets see how Rory's first day of swim went.

Jumping into the Pool

The pool was freezing cold. Rory was already looking for an excuse to get out of taking these lessons. He sat there with his feet dangling in the cool water pretending to hear everything the Flint girl was saying about last night.

In reality I was pretty damn nervous and couldn't believe I was doing this.

As they waited, more and more kids entered the pool. Rory noticed it was nothing but toddlers. Eventually a kid wearing a red swimsuit and blue jacket yelled out, "All right, guys, we are about to get started with little aqua tots beginners class!"

Holy fuck. Could this get anymore embarrassing? This girl, possibly 14 or 15 years old, is in charge of teaching me to swim alongside a pool full of toddlers and babies.

At that point Rory made his mind up to bail on baby camp. He hopped out the pool and began walking toward his towel.

The young girl yelled, "Mr. Thomas! Mr. Thomas!"

Rory kept walking and then realized she was calling him Mr. Thomas.

"Oh, no, you probably have me mistaken for someone else. My name is Rory Powers. I accidentally came here."

Confused, the young girl replied, "Oh, I'm sorry. I just assumed you had the same last name as your wife. She told me to make sure I didn't let you run off."

Damn it. This Flint girl is a thorn even when she's not around.

"Yeah, I think I should hold out for the older people's class."

"Well, actually Mr. Powers, this is probably your best place to start. Not only do you get the basics but you also gain the inspiration of seeing how fearless children can be. It may spark something in you. Adults are limited by logic whereas kids have limitless imagination.

Just hop in and give it a go. Try your best to look at yourself as a beginner just as the children are, instead of looking at the age difference. No matter what the number behind your ID says, you are still a beginner and you should give yourself ultimate permission to be a child again."

Am I being schooled by a 15-year-old? What the hell.

"Okay, these are babies, though. How can an adult learn the same way as babies who can't even walk or talk?"

"It's actually really simple. Once you get in the pool, I'll begin."

Just as Rory was getting ready to walk back toward the pool, The Flint Girl yelled out, "Just get in the pool Rory!!"

"Okay! I just had a couple questions before we started." Rory yelled back.

The young swim coach smiled as Rory hopped in.

Just Begin

Often people want to be in charge of the way they are seen in the eyes of others. There is something extremely nerve wracking about just beginning. The first time doing anything is the scariest.

Early in the book, I explained how Rory learned to ride his bike without training wheels. Well, at the younger ages, most of us have no reputation—or, dare I say, an ego that we fear bruising. It's for that reason we see kids clearing tremendous hurdles at that age span. However, as we age and develop into adults with identities, so does the ego. One of the greatest things you can do for yourself is to continue to put yourself into positions where you must set your ego aside. Within your personal development, you will have days and tasks where everything goes well and you'll also have days where nothing you do goes quite right. Rory is about to experience a lesson that will change his perspective on life forever.

Pool Time

"Okay guys, on the count of three I want you to begin blowing bubbles in the water."

MANNN!!!! I'm not doing this.

Rory stood six feet tall in the pool just four feet deep, staring, surrounded by five other infants and toddlers as their moms placed their children's mouths in the water to begin blowing bubbles as instructed. Flint Girl nudged him.

"Stop being rude. Just do what she asks. It's only a 30-minute lesson, it won't hurt you to participate."

With a side-eyed glare at the Flint Girl, Rory squatted down and began blowing bubbles with the rest of his classmates.

The swim coach yelled, "Okay, great job everyone. Next we are going to go underwater. If your child gets a little anxious, don't worry, it's completely normal. Each time they go under they will become more and more comfortable."

The swim coached looked around to assure that everyone was ready "One...two...three...Dip!"

Each parent went under with their baby and stood back up quickly to celebrate.

"Great job, guys!"

All the kids seemed to get a laugh out of the excitement. Rory, however, needed to climb out the pool.

"Are you okay, Rory?!" yelled the coach

"*Yes, I'm fine. I just got water in my nose and eyes. Give me a second.*"

"Oh yeah, that stings a bit, but if it helps I have a pair of goggles over there you can use."

"*No, that's okay,*" Rory laughed in disbelief. "*I don't need goggles for this class. Just blowing my nose really quick then I'm hopping back in.*"

As Rory hopped back in, the coach took them through four more dunks, each time a second longer than the one before.

My eyes are on fire but I refuse to let these babies handle it and I can't.

"Okay guys, next we are going to put it all together. We are going to dip under water and begin blowing bubbles a second or so. Start blowing bubbles with their head above water first."

The coach made her way over to Rory.

"Hey, are you good? You can go right under when I count to three instead of staying above."

"Okay, yep, I'll do that."

Just as she got to three, Rory submerged his head completely in the water and tried to blow bubbles.

Oh my god, what is happening? I can't see or hear anything. I can't blow bubbles…My heart, I can feel it beating…Oh my god, I have to go back up. I can't stand up. I keep slipping.

"Rory! Rory! It's okay. It's okay. Good job."

"Holy sheeezus that was crazy!!!!" Rory yelled.

He was wrapped around the young swim coach's leg like a baby begging his mom to stay. Everyone in the pool was looking at the two of them.

"Just breathe. You did really well. You just got a little anxious when you went under. That's completely normal."

"I couldn't see anything or hear anything. I couldn't even remember how to blow bubbles. It was like I shut down. That was a crazy feeling that I don't think I've ever felt before."

"Yes, it is very common for a person just learning to swim to become anxious in the process."

Rory backed up from the young coach in embarrassment.

"Sorry about grabbing your leg. I was looking for anything I could to latch onto."

"Oh no worries, it's completely innocent."

"So how do I get over the anxiety? I never even realized I had it."

"Oh, that's easy. First understand I am not saying you have anxiety, I'm saying you had an anxious moment. The way you get through it is simple. You take a deep breath and you go down again."

"Just go back and do the same thing that gave me anxiety the first time?"

"Yep! You have to face your fear of the water in order to overcome the thoughts. That's all they are, are thoughts. You weren't drowning, you actually could have stood up if you didn't let the totality of the moment overwhelm you. This time as you go under, instead of looking at everything, pay attention to each thing as its own individual entity."

"What do you mean?"

"I mean I want you to take a deep breath and as you go under and observe the sounds in your ear. Identify what that is instead of saying you can't hear. You cannot hear what you want to hear, but you can in fact hear. You'll realize it's water you hear. You said that you couldn't see, but if you open your eyes, you will see its water in front of you. Relax your face and trust that when you need air, all you have to do is stand up and get it. Lastly, if you feel your heart beating, appreciate that. It means you are still alive," she said as she laughed.

"Then if you feel good to go, start blowing bubbles. The main thing is you want to remain calm in the water. It can tell when you are distraught. With every angry swipe in the water, more aggressive waves occur. The more energy you exert, the closer you are to your greatest fear of drowning. Instead of fighting the external thing, deal with the internal force, which is you."

"See the water. Feel the water. Hear the water. Recognize that it is just water. Keep practicing, you'll be amazed at how fast you are able to learn once you get over the discomfort."

Rory finished out the session. Each tip she gave him, he began instilling immediately. He stayed an extra 30 minutes over going underwater, repeating the words of his wise young coach.

See the water. Feel the water. Hear the water. It's just water. Be the observer of the waves until they stop and become calm.

As he held his breath underwater, he had become so calm that he could look up and see the young coach standing above, looking at him with a smile. He hopped up.

"I calmed down and the waves went away! I could see you crystal clear!"

"Yes! That's exactly what I wanted you to see! So often we exert so much unnecessary energy that causes more frustration than help. Slow down and see what is instead of worrying about what isn't. It's just water."

"This really was a good class. I hate that I am leaving tomorrow."

"Oh absolutely. I think you have enough to play around with for now. When you get home, keep practicing and have fun with it. Remember to not take yourself too seriously. Practice over perfection. Everyone learns differently, so practice until you figure out your way."

Do Not Sweat Over the Words

Rory fear was not the water it was what can happen in the water. He feared drowning. As his coach asked him to look at the water for what it is, it didn't overwhelm him as much. Rory was afraid of the unknown; he was unable to identify what he was seeing or feeling, which caused a panic. The unknown path is typically when worries and doubts creep in. When he broke his fear into small pieces the task became attainable. He was asked to observe each element of being in water, the sound, the look, and the feel, all as abstract things that did not define him. This is the master key to your liberation. Look at each task for what it is,break them into chunks and take a deep breath if the big picture overwhelms you. The most important thing is to keep going forward. Right on the other side of discomfort is growth..

The way you do anything is the way you do everything. I have a feeling the practice over perfection mindset he learned in swim class will come back really soon to help him.

Its Yoga Time!

Once Rory finally got out of the pool, Flint Girl sat on a pool chair smiling in satisfaction.

"You enjoyed it, didn't you?"

"Yeah, I did. She was good. I'm ready to conquer the world! I'm about to go jump in the ocean!! AHHHHHH!!!! I had never been underwater like that, but after being in there a minute, I was good. I feel lighter... like I can do anything!"

"Slow down, caveman. Didn't you say you had a yoga class to be at this morning too?"

"Shoot, yes, what time is it?!"

"It's 10:45"

"Fawk! I'm supposed to be there at 11!"

By the time Rory made it to the yoga studio, they had already started. The thin yoga lady was not letting him leave without an experience this time.

"Rory, you are late for this class, but I have something even better that you are right on time for. We have a Buddhist meditation teacher in the small room."

Excited for the experience, Rory lit up.

This was already feeling like some exotic shit. I walked in, and the smell of sandalwood was in the air.

The Yoga Lady sent Rory down the hall leading to the meditation room. Quiet as a mouse, Rory was afraid to walk too loud. He looked around the place for a second. Suddenly two small guys popped out to greet him halfway to the door.

"Hi, can we help you?"

"*Hey, yes I'm here for meditation.*"

"Oh yes, yes. Welcome. Let me get you signed in, place your shoes here."

They were very gracious and chill, no more than five-foot-three in height and wearing orange robes. *I'm getting the real deal,* is all Rory could think.

"After you've signed in, you can follow me."

He escorted Rory to a room that kind of resembled a living room. Nothing extravagant. It was literally just a room with a bunch of cushions. An altar sat at the head of the room with Buddhist artifacts and statues. The sandalwood that Rory could smell was burning at the base of the altar. The individual line of smoke was rising toward the ceiling.

As time went by, one person at a time entered the room. It was a mixture of ages and races. A handful of white guys came in with their own cushion, and they sat right at the front. An Asian lady made her way in and found a spot. I was shocked to see two black ladies come in looking poised and prepared to meditate. I tried to make eye contact with one of the black girls to get the nod of assurance that this place is cool. She didn't even look my way, though. Just as I was getting caught up in scanning the room, a bell went off and the tiny teacher walked in and sat down at the altar.

"Allow your eyes to close and allow what is to be."

I followed his directions and closed my eyes. Forty or fifty minutes went by. No positive words, or even oceanic sounds coming through a speaker. Not much explanation. Just a lot of sitting with my breath. I was hoping to get some type of clarity from coming to this space. I wanted to be taught how to put myself in this place of peace.

As the meditation ended, the same bell went off again.

"Open your eyes."

Everyone followed the order. Rory stretched his arms and yawned in relief.

"Does anyone have any questions?"

Oh perfect. He's gonna give the answers.

Rory waited for other people to ask the questions that he was yearning for an answer to, but no one worded it right. They kept giving too much wiggle room for a generic answer. So finally Rory raised his hand.

"What's the purpose of meditation if we are only going to look at things as they are? I'm trying to get rid of all the bad stuff in my head."

"Ah, good question, my friend. The purpose of meditation is to better prepare you for the darkness of life and the lights of life. The hope for everyone's day is that it is always happy and full of bliss. But we all know that life does not work this way. We have rainy, cloudy, sunny, snowy and so many other days. Can you close your eyes and pray that the sun comes out on a rainy day? You can try, but I don't believe you will see much success. The storm passing is out of your control.

Do you think it is logical to stay in the warmth of your home every time it rains or snows? Only come out the days when it's pleasantly to your liking? Once again, you may try with a higher possibility of achievement, but you will have wasted a solid portion of your life hiding from the inevitable changes.

Do you think it is possible to realize the sun rises every day, yet there are some days where it is blocked by the clouds? Have we not found great ways to celebrate the changes of weather? In the fall, we have Halloween and Thanksgiving. As the snow falls, we celebrate its beauty with Christmas. We have learned to adapt to the changes of seasons with grace and acceptance. We have no exact date for snowfall or sunshine, but we are mentally prepared for both.

We do not allow it to control our peace because we have found acceptance in the changes."

"Hmmmm. This makes good sense, but I still want to know how it relates to meditation. What's the umbrella for a rainy day in my life?"

"It's not the rain that you should be seeking to avoid. Yes, you get wet from a rainy day and depending on how you view it, this can be a very gloomy and depressing thing. Yet alternatively, you could look at the rain for what it provides you. It supplies water for the planet and all its resources. It cleanses our bodies. Each drop of rain provides a tranquil experience that is soothing for the soul. It's the perspective of the rain being a thing that works for you."

"So try to convince myself that depression is working for me?"

"Yes, this is it! Yes, my friend, this is a grand idea. However, I wouldn't say "convince" yourself. It's more like trust. Trust that the rainy day also known as depression is in some way nourishing you. We have the benefit of knowing that water and sun are needed for the growth of flowers. History has proven this to be the case. Yet we don't know this to be the truth without anything more than trust. You water a plant and you see nothing instantly. Yet you continue watering and eventually will notice a small bud appear over time.

Meditation acts the same way. You sit and observe your thoughts and feelings the same way you view water and the sun on earth. You trust that the rain in your day is necessary for your growth. You accept that the sunshine in your day may be blocked by clouds some days. Your perspective allows your seeds to bud. The plant of peace acknowledges both the sun and rain as nourishment."

"So you look at yourself as a universe in its own right? The many parts of your body make up the Planet inside of you."

"Yes! I like that. Planet You! Along your lifespan already can you agree you have witnessed constant change within yourself?"

"Yes, of course."

"Precisely, all of us can say we have witnessed change in ourselves at the grossest level, from a child to an adult. But there is more change happening within us that we don't realize. We ignore the subtle changes or fail to recognize the changes within us. Most only become aware of an issue after it has snowballed into a problem."

The meditation teacher looked across the room to see if anyone could agree with his sentiment. A guy in the front lifted his hand.

"Basically there has to be some combination of warm and cold weather pressure that causes the storm."

"Yes, exactly. Often this pressure is not realized by the common person until the storm materializes. Weather forecasters make a living watching the pressure of the air and preparing people for the storms to come. This in turn has saved countless lives. Can you imagine a life where you did not know the weather in advance? Imagine being at home one minute and then the next a massive tornado comes in and wipes out the community."

Well this, my friend, is what we do in meditation. In meditation we act as forecasters. Observing the warm and cold pressures as they formulate. This diffuses the storm from tearing through. Just like a forecaster can't prevent a storm, meditation doesn't prevent anger or sorrow. Mediation allows you the space to observe and prepare for what you see coming. This allows you to feel the highs and lows of life without suffering. We observe the good and bad the same way. This leads to a stress free lifestyle as we are prepared for the storms that are sure to come. This ability to witness the changing without attachment stops the chain of dangerous reactions."

"Whoa! I had never had it explained to me this way. So trying to clear my mind is not the goal? Inhale positive, exhale negative? Inhale the roses, exhale the bad stuff. You ever heard of that?"

Laughing now, the teacher said, "I wish we could control negative and positive in such a way that it resembles a booger being blown out."

Laughter broke out.

"The mind wants to stay busy, and often it's the negative that garners the most attention, so the mind stays there. You must always remember that the mind is a tool that is not you. As long as you can remember that you are not your thoughts, you are not your mind, you will remain in control and peace will begin."

Rory left this meditation with a sense of enlightenment that he had never experienced. The meditation itself didn't give many results, but the talk had. In fact, the talk now made the meditation a lot better.

You are not your thoughts. Observe the thoughts. Ride the waves of the thoughts but do not define yourself by these thoughts.

The goal and aim is always to be the observer. To be the forecaster that tells you what the weather is before it comes. The work in meditation prepares you for life outside of meditation.

Practice the Mindset

In 2009 during the Inauguration Ball, the Obamas were to have their first dance in the White House. Billions of people across the world had their eyes glued to the TV screen as the first black couple entered the White House in its highest seat. With what I'm sure was the highest level of expectation in U.S history, the pressure was on the Obamas and this first dance. I assumed they'd hire some highly esteemed dance choreographer to prepare them. Instead, Barack came out with the stiffest two-step dance, mixed with a grin and a couple spins of Michelle. Then the dance was over. It wasn't the extravagant dance I was expecting, but for some reason it didn't seem to matter. No one spoke of a lack of rhythm or showed concern with how his hips swayed. Is it possible that the magnitude of the circumstances was greater than the dance itself, or could it have been that the joy of dancing didn't need to be measured by good or bad? A few years later in yoga teacher training, I would receive my answer.

In 2013 my teacher Jonny was leading us through a class, and midway through he had us break into a dance session. Everyone was dancing, including Jonny. I held back, sticking to a basic cool-ass head bop. After the class, one of my classmates jokingly teased Jonny about "not knowing how to dance." His response was the golden key to my liberation. With a confused face, he replied, "Everyone can dance." This response was instinctive for him but soul piercing for me. I played it back in my head constantly until it turned into a motto. Everyone can dance. Standing up to speak in front of a crowd: "Everyone can dance." Front row in the yoga class, even though I struggle with poses: "Everyone can dance." Standing up for what you believe, even if the majority doesn't agree: Yes, you can fucking dance!

The good versus bad has been a broken system for years. Whoever made the measuring stick must not have known that the President of the United States of America would one day dance without a care about a scale of good versus bad. Or that a yogi would do a dance in the midst of a yoga class that would unleash the soul of another. Tell me, why should anything else be measured on a scale? If your soul yearns, then move toward it. For this reason, I scream, let the people dance. Let your soul dance. Take off the mask and dance, dance, dance.

Rory Finally Takes Class

After meditation, the thin yoga lady greeted Rory with a huge smile.

"Are you ready for yoga now? I had a talk with the teacher, and they said you can join in with no experience. They will give you some basics to start off with. This is Mysore style yoga, so everyone will be doing their own thing. Do your best to focus on you. Do not fall into the trap of matching other people's practice."

"Do you really think I can handle an advanced class with no experience?"

"I do."

The thin yoga lady smiled and handed him a yoga mat and towel.

Without hesitation, Rory took the mat and placed his shoes by the door. He slowly walked into the smoldering hot room where 30 or 40 yogis were all doing their own thing. It was mat to mat and no visible space. Just as Rory went to turn around, he was waved down by a guy with long, dark hair and a Hawaiian-looking skin tone. His tattoos were amazing as his chiseled muscles glazed of sweat. His smile was welcoming as he quickly rolled his mat and signaled for Rory to take his vacated space.

Without pause, Rory rushed over, took the space and began touching his toes. Then he twisted to the right and once again to the left. Just as he was out of things to do, a voice came from behind.

"You must be Rory. You ready to Rock and Roll?"

"Yessir!" Rory replied.

Rory turned around to put a face to the cool voice. It was a slim, younger white guy. He had a smile that made it calming.

"All right, so I'm gonna speak low so that I don't disturb anyone else's practice, but today I'm gonna guide you through a basic Ashtanga class. We will see how much you can handle and go from there."

Just like that, Rory was off into his first yoga class.

Time to Fly Out

After class, Rory glowed in sweat and amazement.

"You killed that bro. How do you feel?"

"I feel great! I never tried anything even close to that before. It was like a full blown workout, while stretching."

"Yeah, man, welcome to Ashtanga Yoga. You get strength, flexibility and so much more with this style. I'll give you a couple links for you to read more about the practice while you are on the plane."

"Plane! Oh shoot, I have to go!"

Rory darted out. He had an hour before his flight was set to board. Heading toward the hotel to get his bags, he was able to check out and hop in his rental car. He was making perfect timing. He looked at his phone, Flint Girl had called him five times and sent three text messages. The last one read, "Well, I hope you have a safe flight! I know you have to board soon. You could have at least said bye."

Rory decided to give her a call as he drove to the airport.

"Don't come calling me now. You're back in Detroit now."

"No, I'm actually speeding to the airport. I did a dope yoga and meditation classes, I completely lost track of time."

"Well go ahead and enjoy your flight. I didn't want anything. Just saying bye."

"You sound a little hurt you didn't get to see your boy before he left."

"Shut up! I'm not hurt. I did enjoy your company, though. Flint is only a couple hours away from Detroit. Maybe I'll slide over to check you out someday."

"Yes definitely. You're cool as fuck!FUUCCK!"

Just as Rory was getting off the phone. He ran into traffic.

"What?! What happened?"

"I was making great time, and now there's traffic."

"Oh dang. It'll probably clear out. How much time do you have?"

"I hope so. I still have about 35 minutes left, and I don't have to check a bag. I should be good."

The traffic eventually cleared out. Rory had 15 minutes to spare. He forgot the rental car he was driving had to go back. That process would eat up his remaining time. As he sprinted to the gate, the attendants informed him that the doors had closed 20 minutes ago. Rory had missed his flight, with no other flights until the next morning.

Chapter 19: 12 More Hours

SOUTH BEACH HAD been so good to Rory. He had discovered the power of purpose in life, learned the importance of eating foods that nourish the soul, even learned to sit through discomfort while learning to swim, meditate and practice yoga. His greatest gift from this birthday was the trust he'd found in sharing his feelings. It wasn't the worst of all scenarios in the world to spend a few more hours in Miami. His first call was Flint Girl.

"You missed your flight, didn't you?" She readily answered the phone.

"*Yep.*"

"Damn, I was hoping you made it. When is the next flight out? My plane leaves at 9pm tonight, maybe you can get on that one."

"*No, they told me they didn't have anything until the morning.*"

"Yikes, well you may as well come kick it with me until you figure out what you're going to do."

Rory headed right back out to get as much time with Flint Girl as he could. He was starting to fall for her sassy company.

As the taxi pulled up to the swank hotel, Rory got out with a sigh of relief. Previously Rory would have deemed missing his flight as a sign of a bad day raining on his parade. Not today, though. Rory didn't view it as bad or good. He simply accepted that he'd missed his flight and another was sure to come.

Maybe this was a result of his talking with the meditation guy or his desire to see the Flint Girl again. Either way, there had been a shift in perspective.

It had become evident that he was going to need a hotel room one more night, so before calling he decided to check availability. To his surprise, Flint Girl was at the desk talking to the receptionist.

"I wanted to see if I could extend my stay to the morning. My flight was delayed a few hours."

She looked back and realized Rory was there. She winked and signaled for him to stay back. Minutes later, she pushed her baby in a stroller towards Rory with a big smile on her face.

"I got you a room for the night."

"What?! Really? You didn't have to buy me a room, I was going to get one."

"I didn't say I bought you anything, are you crazy?" she laughed. "I told them my flight was delayed and brought up the ants that were in the room. They gave me the extension for free." She laughed even harder.

"Oh, well let me shut up."

"Exactly. I need to pack before I am like you and miss my flight. You can bring your little backpack with you, Mr. No Luggage."

Rory and Flint Girl made their way to the room. They had a chemistry that seemed like they had known each other for years instead of two days. As she packed her bags, they laughed and shared story after story. The baby had fallen asleep as soon as they got into the air conditioned room.

"So what are you gonna do when I leave? I only have about an hour before I have to leave. Then you're gonna be alone again."

"I'll probably just lay here and fantasize about you being here to boss me around."

As Rory laughed, Flint Girl walked toward him, standing between his legs as he sat in a chair.

"You don't like when I'm bossy, baby? You want me to talk like the rest of these little girls out here?" She was teasing him with her tone, but this was the closest they had gotten since meeting.

Rory looked up at her as she stood over him.

"Nah, I like bossy a little bit. But know that I'm still a man."

As Rory stood up, Flint Girl wrapped her arms around him. Rory pulled her in from her low back as they met by the lips. Feverishly, they attacked each other like the attraction had reached a boiling point.

Rory's hands went from her back to cuffing her butt. She slid her hands under his shirt as ran her nails across his spine. Lifted his shirt as she began kissing the rips of Rory's six-pack chiseled abs. He made his hands up the back of her shirt to pop the bra holding her voluptuous breasts. Her hand slid towards the front of his pants. She went to fish out the size of Rory's rod until a scream stopped everything.

"Oh baby! What's wrong? I'm right here."

As Flint Girl strapped her bra back and straightened her pants, she grabbed her baby and began rocking him. In disbelief, Rory fell back into the chair.

Unbelievable. He was the calmest baby for two days straight and now as soon as mommy bout to get some action, he turns into a baby cock blocker.

"You good over there, Rory?" she asked with a smirk.

"Ummm yes I'm good. I think."

"We weren't going any further than that anyway, so don't be too disappointed."

They both laughed but knew they had opened up a can of worms that wouldn't end here.

The next morning, Rory woke up alone to the sun rising. He decided to spend his last morning at the beach watching the sun rise again. This time he wanted to practice what he'd learned.

As he approached the beach, he noticed kids playing and smiled. The sand was full of debris, and he kicked it aside to clear him a space to sit. He watched the ocean waves crash at different levels but in perfect sync. He could hear the seagulls screech and the wind blowing. It was like a beautiful chorus. The sun peeked in and out from behind the clouds. He went from hot to cold as the sun blazed his skin and cooled as the sun hid. Rory sat with the elements. His thoughts went to his mom as he looked at the clouds. He began crying. A kid nearby noticed.

"Are you okay?"

"*Yep, thanks kid. I'm just enjoying the moment.*" Rory smiled and allowed the sun to dry his tears.

"But you're crying. I only cry when I am sad," the kid said in confusion.

"*Yep, me too. I cry when I'm sad and that's okay. It took me a long time to realize there's nothing wrong with being sad or crying.*"

"My dad tells me to have a moment, not a sad day."

"*You have a great dad, kid.*"

Life is about flow. Part of the flow is the moments where our thoughts and feelings change just as much as nature. If you watch closely, you'll find beauty in all of it. The TRAP that we live in starts and stops in our minds. If we can change the way we perceive the things that shape us, then we in fact can find the key to a life of liberation. This involves trusting that today is happening for you. It requires revealing your stories, feelings and thoughts but relinquishing your attachment to them. Accepting what you see as you reveal but setting an aim toward the image you desire to reach. You strive toward the aims with an approach of practice over perfection as we know, nobody is perfect nor should they try to be. Life is flow. Practice it in everything you do, and you will discover you were never trapped in the first place.

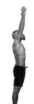

**1.INHALE> Lift both arms,
gaze past the fingertips.**
Note: You want to reach your arms up as high as you can get full extension. Be sure to inhale as you are reaching.

**2. EXHALE> forward fold at the waist,
dropping the crown of your head.
(UTTANASANA)**
Note:The focus should be on folding from the waist.

**3. INHALE> Look up for breath, gaze past 3rd
eye (up) (ARDHA UTTANASANA)**
Note:Don't skip this pose

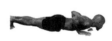

**4. EXHALE> Lower to the bottom of a
pushup, gaze beyond tip of nose
(CHATURANGA DANDASANA)**

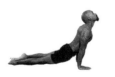

**5. INHALE> Heart goes up,roll onto tops of
feet, bring , gaze past 3rd eye (up) (URDHVA
MUKHA SVANASANA) UPWARD DOG**
NOTE: Press chest forward to avoid dumping into low back.

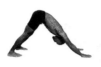

6. EXHALE> Curl your toes , raise hips and drop ypur head, gaze at the navel or through the legs, take 5 breaths (ADHO MUKHA SVANASANA) DOWNWARD DOG

NOTE:Feet shoulder width. If this is too exhausting come to your knees but do not stop.You are building your practice.

7. INHALE> Look up for breath, gaze past 3rd eye (up) (ARDHA UTTANASANA)

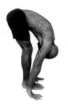

8. EXHALE> forward fold at the waist, dropping the crown of your head. (UTTANASANA)

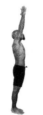

9. INHALE> Lift both arms, gaze past the fingertips.

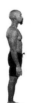

10. EXHALE> hands at side or the heart center, gaze beyond tip of nose. *Finish in sama-sthiti*

REPEAT 5 ROUNDS. TURN THE MUSIC UP!

SURYA NAMASKARA B

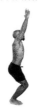

1. INHALE> Lift your arms, (with knees bent) gaze past fingertips (UTKATASANA) CHAIR POSE

2. EXHALE> forward fold at the waist, dropping the crown of your head. (UTTANASANA)

3. INHALE> Look up for breath, gaze past 3rd eye (up) (ARDHA UTTANASANA) (ARDHA UTTANASANA)

4. EXHALE> Lower to the bottom of a pushup, gaze beyond tip of nose (CHATURANGA DANDASANA)

5. INHALE> Heart goes up,roll onto tops of feet, bring , gaze past 3rd eye (up) UPWARD DOG
NOTE: Take a big inhale here the next pose will require a long exhale.

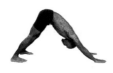

6. EXHALE> Curl toes under, raise hips for
DOWNWARD DOG, immediately step the right
foot forward, left foot turns out.
Note: This is may take time to get use to but its a
long exhale as you step through for Warrior A.

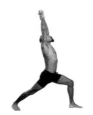

6B. INHALE> Lift arms, gaze past fingertips
(VIRABHADRASANA A) WARRIOR A
NOTE: Notice most of the pose was done during
the prior step.

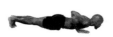

7. EXHALE> Lower to the bottom of a pushup,
gaze beyond tip of nose (CHATURANGA
DANDASANA)

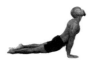

8. INHALE> Lift your heart for UPWARD DOG
(ARDHVA MUKHA SVANASANA)

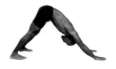

9A. EXHALE> Curl toes under, raise hips for
DOWNWARD DOG, immediately step the left
foot forward, right foot turns out.
Note: This is may take time to get use to but its a
long exhale as you step through for Warrior A.

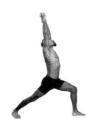

9B. INHALE> Lift arms, gaze past fingertips (VIRABHADRASANA A) WARRIOR A NOTE: Notice most of the pose was done during the prior step. (VIRABHADRASANA A)

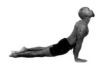

10. EXHALE> Lower to the bottom of a pushup, gaze beyond tip of nose (CHATURANGA DANDASANA)

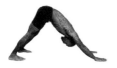

11. INHALE> Lift your heart for UPWARD DOG (ARDHVA MUKHA SVANASANA)

12. EXHALE>Curl toes under, raise hips for DOWNWARD DOG take 5 breaths here (ADHA MUKHA SVANASANA)

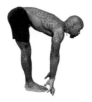

13. INHALE> look up for breath

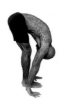

**14. EXHALE> Forward Fold
(UTTANASANA)**

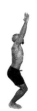

**15. INHALE> Knees bent, arms and torso rise up,
gaze past thumbs
(UTKATASANA) CHAIR POSE**

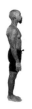

**16. EXHALE> straighten legs, hands at side or to
heart center, gaze beyond tip of nose**

Finish in sama-sthiti

REPEAT 5 ROUNDS. TURN THE
MUSIC UP!

Figure 1

1. PADANGUSTHASANA

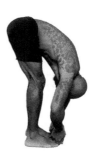

INHALE> hop or step feet 6 to 8 inches apart
    EXHALE> hands to hips
INHALE> look up and bend back slightly
    EXHALE> fold forward... "peace fingers" to big toes
INHALE> look up for breath
    EXHALE> fold fowrad... gaze to navel or between
legs... 5 breaths

Figure 2

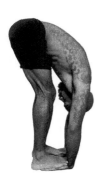

2. PADAHASTASANA

INHALE> Look up halfway past 3rd eye
  EXHALE> release toes... sliding palms of hands under soles
                 of feet/toes to wrist
INHALE> look up
    EXHALE> fold forward... Gaze between legs...chest to
                 thighs... 5 breaths
INHALE> Look up past 3rd eye
    EXHALE> hands to hips
INHALE> come all the way up to standing
    EXHALE> step or hop feet together... palms touch at
              heart center... gaze off tip of nose.

Finish in sama-sthiti

3. UTTHITA TRIKONASANA (Trianagle Pose0
Begin in sama-sthiti

INHALE> step out to the right,facing the long
edge of your mat feet about 4 feet apart, right
foot out...arms to a "T"
    EXHALE> reach out over the right hip and
then bring right hand to right first toe, ankle, or
shin
INHALE> stretch up through left fingertips...
gaze up past left hand.... 5 breaths
    EXHALE> look down
INAHLE> come up to strong "T" and change
sides
    EXHALE> reaching out over left hip, bring
left hand to left frist toe, ankle, or shin
INHALE> stretch up through right fingertips...
gaze up past right hand... 5 breaths
    EXHALE> look down
INHALE> come back up to "T"

Figure 3

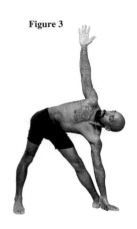

4. PARIVRTTA TRIKONASANA (Revolve Triangle Pose)

INHALE> switching feet again to right... turning hips to
follow, extending left arm up
    EXHALE> left hand plants down inside or outside
right foot
INHALE> lift right arm to the sky... gaze follows right
hand... heart open ... 5 breaths
    EXHALE> look down
INHALE> come up to strong "T"... switch feet, turning
hips to left, extending right arm up
    EXHALE> right hand plants down besides left foot
INHALE> lift left arm to the sky... gaze follows left
hand... heart is open... 5 breaths
    EXHALE> look down
INHALE> come up to strong "T"
    EXHALE> close pose by stepping feet together at
front of the mat... palms touch at heart center

sama-sthiti

Figure 4

5. UTTHITA PARSVAKONASANA (Side Angle Pose)

INHALE>step out to the right about 5 feet... right foot turned out... arms to a T

EXHALE> bend 90 degrees into the right knee... place right hand down outside right foot or place forearm on thigh

INHALE>. stretch left arm over head (bicep to ear) ... left nipple turns out... gaze past left hand... take 5 breaths

EXHALE>look down

INHALE> come up to T and change sides

EXHALE> bend into the left knee 90 degrees... place left hand down outside left foot or place forearm on thigh

INHALE> stretch arm over head ... right nipple turns up... gaze past right fingertips... 5 breaths

EXHALE> look down

INHALE> back up to T... changing sides

EXHALE> palms come together at heart center

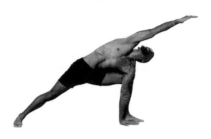

Figure 5

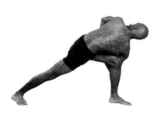

Figure 6

6. PARIVTTA PARSVAKONASANA

INHALE> changing sides... rotating hips to the right

EXHALE> as you lunge into the right knee, palms at prayer, hook left elbow outside right knee

INHALE> twisting, lifting heart in line with the hands... gaze up over the right shoulder... hold 5 breaths

EXHALE> look down

INHALE> back up to strong T... change sides... rotate hips to the left

EXHALE> as you lunge into the left knee, palms at prayer, hook right elbow outside left lunging knee

INHALE> twisting, lifting heart in line with hands... gaze up over the left shoulder... hold 5 breaths

EXHALE> look down

INHALE> come up to strong T

EXHALE> step feet through at top of mat... sama-sthiti

7. PRASARITA PADOTTANASANA A

INHALE> step out to the right about 5 feet. arms to a T
EXHALE> fold forward... plant hands about 1 foot apart in line with heels
INHALE> lift chest up halfway... look past 3rd eye
EXHALE> fold in... crown of head reaching toward floor as chin tucks... gaze between the legs... hold 5 breaths
INHALE> look up
EXHALE> hands to hips
INHALE> hands on hips coming all the way up
EXHALE> root feet

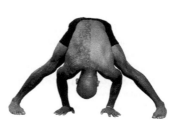

Figure 7

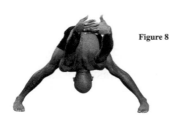

Figure 8

8. PRASARITA PADOTTANASANA C

INHALE> bring arms to T
EXHALE> Interlace fingers behind hips
INHALE> bend back from the heart... hands draw down below tailbone
EXHALE> fold forward... hands still clasped, moving away from low back... gaze between legs... chin tucks... hold 5 breaths
INHALE> come all the way up
EXHALE> hand to hips... root feet.

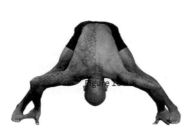

10. PRASARITA PADOTTANASANA D

INHALE> arms to T
EXHALE> fold forward and bind big toes
INHALE> lift heart and gaze past 3rd eye
EXHALE> fold in deep... elbows splay out... crown of head toward floor
INHALE> look up
EXHALE>Place hands on the floor
INHALE>Look up

Figure 11

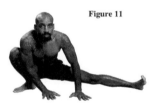

11.EXHALE> side bend into right knee
INHALE> back to center
EXHALE> Side bend into the left knee
Repeat 5 Times

Figure 12

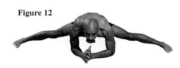

12.Samakonasana (Center Splits)
INHALE> Stop in the center
EXHALE> Heel toe your feet apart until
you find your limit....Hold for 5 breaths

Figure 13

13.Hanumanasana>(Front Splits Pose)
INHALE>Look up
EXHALE>Step your right leg out in front and straighten it ... Hold 5
Breaths
INHALE> LOOK UP
EXHALE> CHANGE SIDES Front splits to the left...Hold 5 Breaths
INHALE>Standing up Strong T
EXHALE>Close it out at the top of the mat

11. PARSVOTTANASANA
begin in sama-sthiti

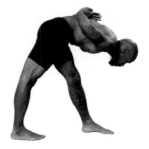

Figure 11

INHALE> step out to the right about 2 to 3 feet all ten toes face the back of the mat.

EXHALE> bring palms together behind back... reverse namaste

INHALE> lift heart... look up

EXHALE> lead with your heart as your fold over right leg... gaze to shin or head to knee... hold for 5 breaths

INHALE> come up and change sides... turning feet and hips to the left

EXHALE> adjust hands... wiggle them up between shoulder blades

INHALE> lift heart... slight backbend... look up

EXHALE> lead with your heart as you fold over the left leg... gaze to shin... 5 breaths

INHALE> come all the way up... arms to T

EXHALE> come back to sam/sthiti

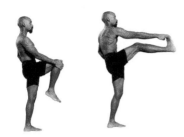

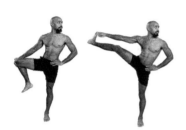

Figure 12-15

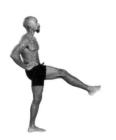

12. UTTHITA HASTA PADANGUSTHASANA A
INHALE> right knee into chest... catch knee with
right hand
EXHALE> catch right first toe with peace fingers
INHALE> extend leg out in front of you... gaze off
tip of nose... hold for 5 breaths

13. UTTHITA HASTA PADANGUSTHASANA B
EXHALE> open up to the right... gaze over the left
shoulder... hips level... 5 breaths

14. UTTHITA HASTA PADANGUSTHASANA C
INHALE> bring leg back through center
EXHALE> catch foot with both hands and hug in...
head to knee
INHALE> keep leg and lift heart

15. UTTHITA HASTA PADANGUSTHASANA D
EXHALE> hands to hips... keeping right leg
extended high in front of you... gaze off tip of nose...
5 breaths
INHALE> lift right foot a bit higher
EXHALE> bring the foot to the floor... change sides

Go through LEFT side A, B, C, & D... finishing D in sama-shiti

16. Vrksasana (Tree Pose) to Natarajasana (Dancer Pose)

INHALE> right foot inside the left leg above or below the knee

EXHALE> Prayer hands to heart center

INHALE> Hands extend up gaze at your fingertips ... 5 breaths

EXHALE> Right hands grabs inside the right foot

INHALE>Left arm extends up

EXHALE> The heart goes forward while right leg goes up... Hold 5 Breaths

INHALE> Stand all the way up keeping the right leg lifted one breath

EXHALE> lower foot to floor... change sides

Go through LEFT side...
finishing in sama-shiti

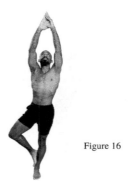

Figure 16

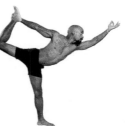

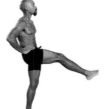

Figure 16

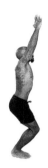

17. UTKATASANA (CHAIR POSE)
Take a FULL VINYASA...just like a Sun Salutation letter A... taking one inhale in downward dog...

EXHALE> float feet between hands and bend knees as you land... big toe kiss
INHALE> sweep arms above head and heart... sitting back
5 breaths
EXHALE> fold over stright legs

18. VIRABHADRASANA A
Take a FULL VINYASA...just like a Sun Salutation letter A... one inhale in downward dog...

EXHALE> down dog... right foot steps up... back heel flat
INHALE> lift your heart... raise arms over head... gaze up... hold for 5 breaths... on the last inhale... straighten the right leg... gaze still up... pivot and turn to the other side
EXHALE> bend left knee deeply... 5 breaths... gaze remains lifted

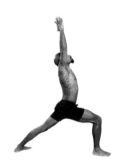

19. VIRABHADRASANA B
EXHALE> with the last exhale on the left side of letter A... open arms to T... square hips to the long edge of the mat... gaze past left hand... 5 breaths
INHALE> straighten left leg and pivot turn to the other side
EXHALE> bend right knee 90 degrees... gaze beyond right fingertips... 5 breaths
INHALE> last inhale very deep
EXHALE> hands surround front right foot

1.VINYASA to seated postures

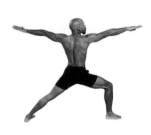

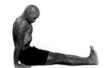

2. DANDASANA
From the down dog in VINYASA from
Virabhadrasana B...

INHALE> hop or step feet 6 to 8 inches apart
EXHALE> jump through to seated and extend
legs... toes point upwards
INHALE> plant hands by hips and sit up tall
EXHALE> tuck chin toward chest.. gaze
downward... hold 5 breaths

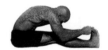

3. PASCHIMOTTANASANA A
INHALE> stretch arms up over head... lift gaze
EXHALE> fold forward... catch first toes
INHALE> lift heart and lengthen... gaze up
EXHALE> fold forward... chest to thighs...
gaze down... 5 breaths

4. PASCHIMOTTANASANA B
INHALE> lift heart... look up
EXHALE> release bind... wrap hands
around outside of feet...
INHALE> lift heart... look up
EXHALE> fold... 5 breaths

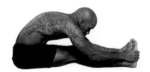

5. PASCHIMOTTANASANA C
Option to clasp wrist

6. PURVOTTANASANA (Reverse Plank)
INHALE> lift heart... look up
EXHALE> release foot or wrist... plant
hands 1 foot behind hips... fingers facing
heels
INHALE> lift up hips to reverse plank...
gaze back...hold 5 breaths
EXHALE> hips down softly

7. JANU SIRSASANA A
From down dog in HALF VINYASA...

EXHALE> coming through to seated...
extended left leg out... bring sole of right
foot to inner left thigh
INHALE> reach arms overhead... look up
EXHALE> fold over left leg... reaching
for foot
INHALE> lift heart for length
EXHALE> fold over left leg... 5 breaths
INHALE> lift heart... look up
EXHALE> release foot... change sides

Repeat on other side...
INHALE>/HALF VINYASA to the next
posture

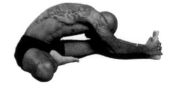

8.&9. MARICHYASANA A & C
From down dog in the HALF VINYASA...

EXHALE> come through to seated... extend both legs out
INHALE> bend right knee
EXHALE> left hand behind your back
INHALE> right hand reaches up
EXHALE> fold inside of the right knee reaching for the left hand behind you... gaze at left toes
INHALE> look up
EXHALE> release bind
INHALE> come up
INHALE> change sides

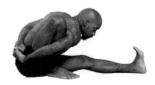

From down dog in the HALF VINYASA...
EXHALE> come through to seated... extend both legs out
INHALE> bend right knee.. plant sole of foot on floor inside left thigh... heel close to hip
EXHALE> place right hand 6 inches behind right hip
INHALE> stretch left arm up... extending through fingertips... lift gaze
EXHALE> hook left elbow outside right knee... twisting to the right... you may bind... gaze over your right shoulder...
INHALE> look forward
EXHALE> unwind arms and extend both legs forward

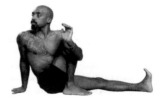

Repeat on other side...
INHALE/HALF VINYASA to next posture

10. NAVASANA (BOAT POSE)

From down dog HALF VINYASA...
EXHALE> come through to seated
INHALE> lift legs to 45 degrees... extend arms forward... hold for 5 breaths
EXHALE> plant hands in front of hips... cross legs
INHALE> bump up... lifting hips, legs, and maybe feet, off the floor

Option: move to the wall for Handstand in between

EXHALE> set bottom back down

Repeat 2 to 4 more times. To finish last one...
INHALE> bump up

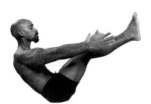

11. BADDHA KONASANA (BOUND ANGLE POSE)

INHALE> come through to seated... bend your knees, place the bottoms of your feet together and bring the heels into the groin... open the feet like a book
EXHALE> lift your chin and look up
INHALE> fold forward keeping your elbows close to the ribs... bring chest toward feet and chin toward the floor... gaze off the tip of your nose... hold for 5 breaths
EXHALE> sit up
INHALE> release
EXHALE/HALF VINYASA to next posture

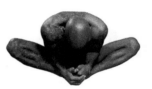

12. UPAVISTHA KONASANA A (SEATED ANGLE POSE)

EXHALE> come through to seated... open your feet to a wide straddle, legs straight and grab your big toes
INHALE> lift halfway... look up
EXHALE> fold forward, take chest and chin to the floor.. gaze at your third eye... hold for 5 breaths

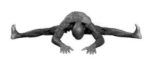

13. URDHVA DHANURASANA (BRIDGE POSE)

EXHALE> come through to lying on your back... walk feet up to hips... arms alongside body

INHALE> lift hips... clasp hands underneath body... roll shoulder blades underneath you... lift chest... chin tucks... 5 breaths [BRIDGE]

EXHALE> come down... place hands beside ears... fingers facing shoulders... preparing for upward bow

14. URDHVA DHANURASANA (WHEEL POSE)

INHALE> press into hands and feet, lifting entire mid body off the floor... working to straighten arms and legs... 5 breaths [WHEEL]

EXHALE> tuck chin to chest... lower body down

Repeat 1 to 3 more times, OPTIONAL BRIDGE OR WHEEL on the last

EXHALE> come down and squeeze knees into chest... hold for few breaths... rocking from side to side

15. PASCHIMOTTANASANA II

From knees hugged into chest

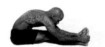

INHALE> rock up to seated and extend legs and reach arms above head

EXHALE> fold forward... catch big toes, feet or wrist hold for 15 breaths

INHALE> lift chest... look up

EXHALE> let go of feet... lie down on back ... extend legs and squeeze together... point toes...

16. SALAMBA SARVANGASANA(Shoulder Stand)

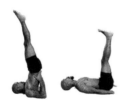

INHALE> lift legs up to a point at the ceiling

EXHALE> swing legs over head or toward the floor... lifting hips over shoulders... place hands on lower back to adjust neck and shoulders

INHALE> extend legs up toward the ceiling... hold for 15 to 25 breaths

17. HALASANA (PLOW POSE)

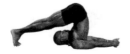

EXHALE> bring legs down behind head to floor if possible... clasp hands behind back.. hold for 5 to 10 breaths

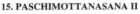

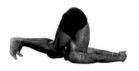

18. KARNAPIDASANA (EAR PRESSUE POSE)
INHALE> bend knees and bring them down towards ears... press
knees to ears if possible... hold for 5 breaths
EXHALE> roll out of the posture to lying on your back with legs
togther and arms extended beside you

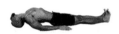

19. MATSYASANA (FISH POSE)
EXHALE> lie flat on your back...
extend legs and point toes...
INHALE> arch your neck and back
bringing the crown of your head to
the floor
HOLD 5 BREATHS

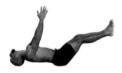

20. UTTANA PADASANA
INHALE> lift legs 45 degrees...
extend them out... same with arms...
placing palms together... hold for 5
breaths
EXHALE> bring arms and legs
down..

21. PADMASANA
INHALE> sit up
EXHALE> place the back of your
hands on your knees, bring your
first finger and thumb together...
tuck chin to chest... look at your
naval... hold for 10 breaths

22. UTPLUTHIH TOLASANA(BREATH OF FIRE)
INHALE> plant hands next to hips, lift up and balance... hold for 108 rounds of Bhastrika Pranayama

Simhasana (Lion's Breath) - 3 Rounds
While still in lotus, roll forward onto knees, exhale through the mouth, making a "ha" sound. As you exhale, open your mouth wide and stick your tongue as far out as possible towards your chin, bringing your drishti towards your third eye as you exhale.

INHALE> roll back bringing forehead to the mat
Repeat for a total of 3 Rounds

Take one final vinyasa thought to savasana

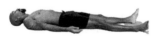

23. SAVASANA I (CORPSE POSE)
EXHALE> legs extend out with ankles mat witdth apart... arms relax to the sides away from hips... palms open... relax body completely... come to natural, normal breath, closed eyes... 5 MINUTES

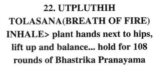

7 DAY YOGI BEGINNERS PLAN

Lightning Source UK Ltd.
Milton Keynes UK
UKHW021002291222
414562UK00009B/1160